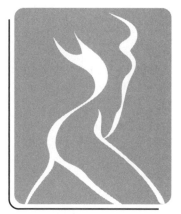

The
SEX DRIVE
Solution
FOR WOMEN

Dr. Jen's Power Plan to Fire Up Your Libido

By Jennifer Landa M.D. and Virginia Hopkins

THE SEX DRIVE SOLUTION FOR WOMEN: DR. JEN'S POWER PLAN TO FIRE UP YOUR LIBIDO

Copyright © 2012 Jennifer Landa M.D., Virginia Hopkins, BodyLogicMD

Atlantic Publishing Group, Inc.
1405 SW 6th Avenue • Ocala, Florida 34471 • Phone 800-814-1132 • Fax 352-622-1875
Website: www.atlantic-pub.com • Email: sales@atlantic-pub.com
SAN Number: 268-1250

Library of Congress Cataloging-in-Publication Data

Landa, Jennifer, 1969-
   The sex drive solution for women : Dr. Jen's power plan to fire up your libido / by Jennifer Landa and Virginia Hopkins.
      p. cm.
   Includes bibliographical references and index.
   ISBN 978-1-60138-718-9 (alk. paper) -- ISBN 1-60138-718-0 (alk. paper)
   1. Sexual desire disorders--Popular works. 2. Women--Sexual behavior--Popular works. 3. Women--Health and hygiene--Popular works. 4. Self-care, Health--Popular works. I. Hopkins, Virginia. II. Title.
   RC560.S46L36 2012
   616.85'8306--dc23
                       2011043737

Printed in the United States

Jennifer Landa, MD, is a brilliant, insightful and caring physician and a leading educator of other doctors.

I would recommend The Sex Drive Solution *to any woman who's looking for the ultimate how-to book on restoring a lost libido. Dr. Landa combines her medical training and patient experiences to cover all the bases, from hormones and hot flashes, to herbal aphrodisiacs and relationship issues.*

> — *Ron Rothenberg, M.D.,* Founder, California HealthSpan Institute
> *Author,* Hormone Optimization in Preventive/Regenerative Medicine

Here's What Dr. Jen's Patients Say...

The balancing of my hormones has improved my sex life tremendously. I wanted sex but wasn't feeling the pleasure of it. Dr. Jen's guidance has brought back the sensations and desire that I felt in my early 20s, and I'm enjoying intimacy with my husband of 25 years even more than I did in our early married years!
— L.J.

I'm a 50-something guy who went to Dr. Jen after seeing the changes my wife experienced after her treatment. I was having trouble sleeping, my brain wasn't as sharp as it had been, and I noticed a decline in my libido. After starting on testosterone, all my symptoms improved immediately! Now I know that the ultimate satisfaction comes when we care enough about our relationship to seek out solutions together.
— J.J.

Thank you for all that you have done for me over the past few years concerning my hormone health after menopause. It has made a world of difference—I sleep well, no more hot flashes or joint pain, and my sex life is
back! It has been four years now, and we still enjoy our intimacy, and that keeps us feeling close to each other as well as keeping us healthy. I thank you and my husband really thanks you!
— E.A.

It took me a few months to really get with the healthy eating and exercise part of your program, but once I did, my whole life started to change in such a great way! I'm a much nicer person to be around and look ten years younger. My family is getting healthier too, and my husband and I love our date nights. Thanks, Dr. Jen, for hanging in there with me.
— L.B.

Dr. Jen, you showed me how to take care of myself, and now I can take care of my family too. I'm sure I was your most frazzled patient ever. At first I just wanted a pill and felt your mindfulness exercises were too "woo woo" for me, but I now I know they saved my marriage. And yes, we did get some sex toys and are having fun again!
— P.G.

This book is for all of the wonderful patients I have been blessed to have the opportunity to help in their journeys toward health, balance and well-being.

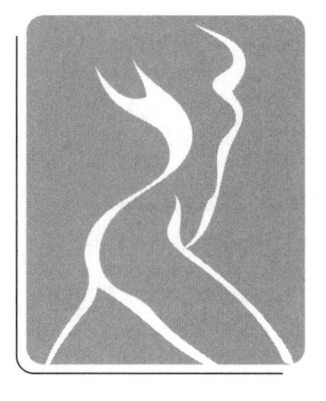

ACKNOWLEDGMENTS

This book would not have been possible without the help of many wonderful people.

First, I'm grateful to the patients who have had the willingness and determination to stick with the Sex Drive Solution program and generously shared their stories with me.

Thank you to my co-author, Virginia Hopkins. Ginny, without your vision, knowledge, experience and wisdom, this book never could have come together as it has. Let's continue the mission to educate women and empower them to help themselves. Melissa Block, your hard work, skill and enthusiasm for the subject made this book possible.

Next, I would like to thank all the folks at BodyLogicMD who have supported me with all of their contributions. Patrick Savage, you are extraordinary in your vision and leadership, which has led BodyLogicMD to become an incredible network of the most highly trained physicians specializing in the field of bioidentical hormone therapy and preventive medicine. Jill Swartz, Marketing VP of BodyLogicMD, has worked tirelessly with her staff to always make everything look and sound great. And Jill, thanks for being there whenever I needed to bounce ideas off you, and thanks for being a good friend. Thanks to the rest of the BLMD team, especially Lisa and Sarah, for all that you do.

Thank you to the crew at Atlantic Publishing. Doug, thanks for your patience with my never-ending questions. Also, thanks for believing in me, this book and the newer areas of medicine we have been exploring. Meg, thank you for your patience with ongoing revisions and changes after changes.

Thank you to Mandy Landa, the best web-chick and sister-in-law I could ask for.

A giant thank you and lots of love to Bonnie Johnson, my office manager, right arm, and amazing friend. You know I could never do any of this without you. I wouldn't want to, and neither would our patients.

Thank you to my long-time friend and "sister," Melissa Gurfein, who is always there to listen, care and share.

I could never have been in the position to help so many without the love and support of my wonderful parents, Lou and Cookie Ziemba, who have always believed in me and told me I could do anything I set my mind to. I love you both. Love and thanks to my brother Rob who always listens without judgment and puts his own unique spin on things for me.

Love, hugs and kisses aplenty to my family. My husband Adam has seen me through it all with love and has been a constant supporter, friend and lover. Thank you for always believing in me, baby, and for helping me get through it all every day. Jonathan and Lexi, thank you for your patience, support, understanding and love, and for trying not to complain too much when Mommy has to work late. I love you all more than words can express.

Finally, I would like to thank you, the reader, who has chosen to take this journey to put the passion and spark back into your sex drive. You will get out of this all that you put into it and more.

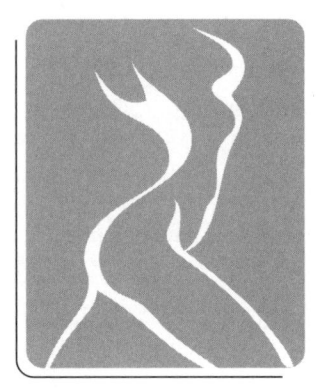

TABLE OF CONTENTS

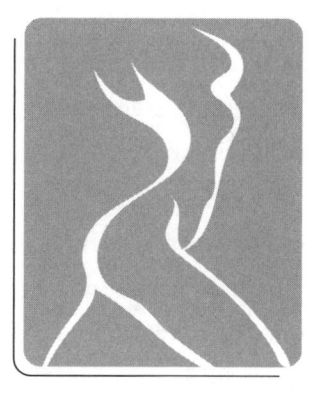

INTRODUCTION

For most doctors, myself included, the best part of seeing patients is helping them feel better. During college I participated in a summer program at a rehab hospital, working with stroke patients when they first came in from an acute care facility and watching them become better through rehab. Sharing in the experience of truly helping patients heal—often dramatically—was intensely rewarding and influenced my decision both to attend medical school and later to focus on women's health with an OB/GYN residency. I knew that the most rewarding path for me as a doctor would be to help women be healthier.

The reality of my first years in practice was different. I was diagnosing women using insurance company codes, prescribing them a drug approved by an insurance company for that diagnosis, and sending them on their way. It was a cookie cutter way of practicing medicine: she's 35, she gets a birth control pill. She's depressed or has mood symptoms, she gets some Zoloft. If she's menopausal or her periods have stopped, she gets PremPro, and then maybe the Zoloft or Prozac on top of that. It was a very formulaic and detached way of practicing medicine.

For example, I had a pill I could prescribe for restless leg syndrome, but I didn't know what to do for adrenal fatigue, which I now know is one of the biggest health issues that women have. I knew almost nothing about hormones. I know that sounds incredible—people think that gynecologists should be hormone experts, but the truth is that in medical school we spent very little time on the biochemistry of hormones. Why would we need to know that when all we needed was the right drug to prescribe? I had never heard of the hormone estriol, which is amazing since it's one of the primary hormones of pregnancy. I didn't know the difference between a progestin and progesterone, or why cortisol levels are so important to a woman in her 40s. Although I didn't know it at the time, I was really practicing in the dark.

Looking for better answers, I attended a large conference where bioidentical hormone therapy (BHRT) was a big topic. After hearing the strong scientific arguments behind BHRT from scientists and success stories from clinicians who were using it for patients every day, I was ready to learn more and soon began to use bioidentical hormones with my patients. They were getting better, they were happy, and I was happy! My practice was rewarding. I signed up for a two-year fellowship affiliated with the American Board of Anti-Aging and Regenerative Medicine and became board certified in that specialty.

Now I'm much more able to get to the root cause of health problems, rather than just putting a Band-Aid® on symptoms. I'm not shooting in the dark, and I'm not exacerbating people's symptoms. In short, I'm happy to be a doctor again.

From early in my clinical practice I saw many women of all ages who had no sex drive. This was an issue I could relate to, because when I was 28 years old I went through a period of time in which I was completely uninterested in sex and didn't care if I ever had sex again! My husband and I will never forget the time we were on a vacation in Colorado and I just wasn't interested in taking advantage of our alone time. He said, "You really don't care at all about sex, do you?"

I replied, "If I'm being dead honest, no. I could go a year and it wouldn't make a difference to me." He eventually said, "All right. I love you, and I'll stay with you, and we'll just have it when we can I guess." This was traumatic for me, like having a dread disease, and I decided, for my husband's sake if not mine, to find out what had happened to my libido. As it turned out, I was on a form of birth control that reduced my sex drive. I was also stressed to the max because I was working 100 hours a week as an OB/GYN resident. No wonder I wasn't interested in sex.

My low libido was a very personal issue and as I successfully worked my way out of it, I found I had some insights to offer my patients. Women talk to each other about problems such as not wanting sex, and they often feel as if there's nobody out there in the medical profession to help them. So word got around, and helping women restore libido became something of a specialty of mine. Now that I know so much more about the biochemistry of libido and have bioidentical hormones in my libido restoration kit, I can truly help most women bring their sex drive back to life.

In this book I'll be delving into the physical side of libido; hormones and pheromones, the G-spot and the clitoris, orgasms and vaginal dryness, masturbation and massage. I'll explain how hormone imbalance, drugs, excess weight and a poor diet can derail your sex life. You'll find out which types of food and exercise are most likely to be helpful and why a nap may be your key to arousal. There is no equivalent of Viagra for women, no one pill or potion, no vitamin or herb, that will magically restore libido. A woman's sex drive is tied to her attention, as well as to her hormones, and her attention is all too often held captive by piles of laundry and dirty dishes. That's why so many women say that one of the sexiest things a man can do is wash the dishes or fold the laundry!

What may be a turn-on to one woman is a turn-off to another, so I'll present a variety of attention-capturing strategies, from yoga, date night and sexy lingerie, to lubricants and bubble baths, meditation and sex toys. In the end, your approach to arousal is going to be intimately, personally yours, but I do have some tried and true approaches to help you get started! What I hope you discover in this book is that cultivating the desire to have sex can be fun and restorative for both you and your partner.

Writing this book is the result of searching for my own answers to the sometimes painful issues surrounding the loss of libido. I have been inspired along the way by so many people, but especially by the patients I have been able to help chart a course back to a healthy sex drive and back to intimacy in their relationships. In addition to better libido, they have seen a return, or sometimes experienced for the first time, the passion and zest that go along with a healthy sex drive. I am thankful every day for the opportunity to help and heal lives. What really makes my day is when patients tell me that they feel better and that I have made a difference in their lives. I cannot see and personally help all who struggle with libido loss and other issues, but I hope that this book can reach out and provide some form of guidance.

Jennifer Landa, M.D.

PART I

The Basics
of Sexuality
and Desire

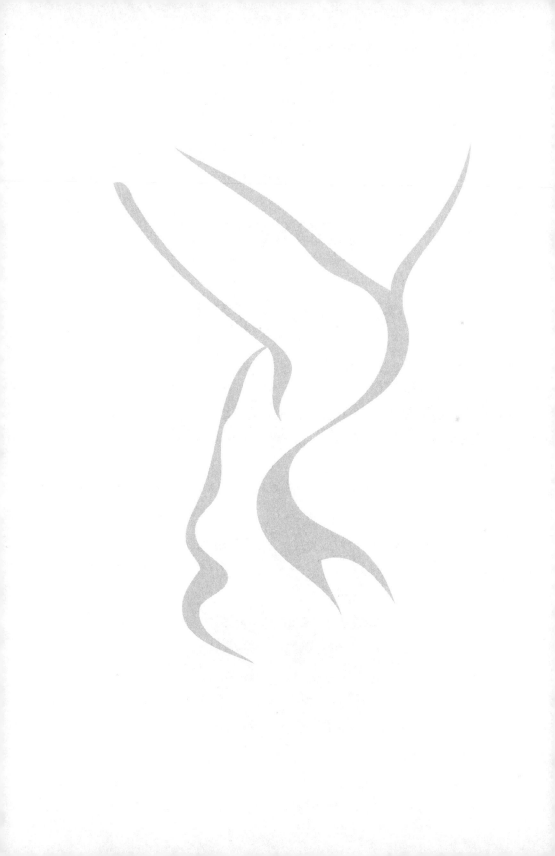

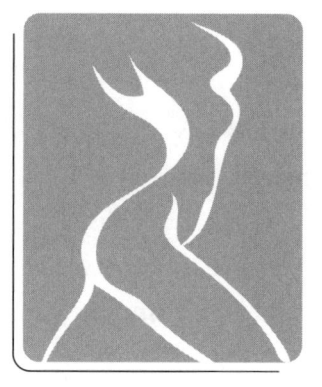

CHAPTER 1

Doctor, I've Lost My Libido!

I t's 11 p.m. and Susan stands in the middle of her living room. The floor is cluttered with toys. The couch is covered with laundry that needs folding and putting away, and the kitchen sink counter overflows with dirty dishes. The sound of canned laughter from a sitcom rerun comes from the TV. Susan has been going nonstop since 5 a.m. that morning and knows that if she sits down to fold the laundry she might not get up again until she awakens at 3 a.m. with a sore neck.

Just then her husband Brad, who has been upstairs on his computer all evening, embraces her from behind and nuzzles her neck suggestively. She can feel the pressure of the gut he's grown over the past few years. His baggy sweats smell like they haven't been washed in months, and his whiskers are scratchy. Just a few years ago, a suggestive nuzzle on the neck would have quickly led to passionate sex on the couch. Tonight Susan has a sudden impulse to jab her elbow into Brad's ribs but instead points to the dirty dishes in the kitchen. "The sexiest thing you could do right now," she says, "is put the dishes in the dishwasher." Brad sighs deeply, then without a word goes back upstairs to the computer.

Susan could be any one of millions of women whose interest in sex with their partner has been replaced by an interest in just getting through the day. She has lost her libido in the dirty dishes, scratchy beard and lack of sleep, and although she occasionally yearns for her days of spontaneous lust for Brad, most of the time she just wishes he would help out more around the house.

The Urge to Merge

Libido is the desire for sex, the physical drive—that feeling like you really *want* it. Libido makes sexual activity feel pleasurable and satisfying. A woman's libido can drop a little bit or fall away completely for many different reasons.

What Susan doesn't realize is that as she approaches the age of 40, her hormone levels are fluctuating, and this, along with the piles of laundry and less-than-romantic husband, adds to her lack of libido.

In our younger years, sex drive has a lot to do with biology and primal urges to reproduce. We naturally create the necessary hormones to ensure that we keep making new human beings. As long as the organism is young and healthy, these drives click in; we want to have sex, and there's a good chance we're going to enjoy it. From a purely physical perspective the primal sex drive becomes less urgent as we enter our 40s and our hormone levels begin to fluctuate. It makes biological sense for sex drive to become less intense as our reproductive years come to an end, but in no way does that mean we have to give up sex!

Restoring libido for a couple like Susan and Brad will be a process, not an event, and will likely involve a physical, mental and emotional makeover for both partners. This may sound like a big job, but I'm going to show you how it can be a fun, rewarding journey that can lead to a more rewarding sex life and a more intimate relationship with your partner.

One in three women (at least) has lost her libido

If you are a female over the age of 30, have low libido, and feel unhappy about it, you have plenty of company. According to current research on American women, about 40 percent of us over the age of 30 have "impaired sexual response." Twenty percent of women with impaired sexual response say that this is a source of significant distress.

According to Emily and Barry McCarthy's book, *Rekindling Desire: A Step-By-Step Program to Help Low-Sex and No-Sex Marriages*, (Brunner-Routledge 2003), "The adage in sex therapy is that when sexuality goes well, it is a positive, integral but not major component—adding 15 to 20 percent to marital vitality and satisfaction. However, when sexuality is dysfunctional or nonexistent, it assumes an inordinately powerful role, 50 to 70 percent, robbing the marriage of intimacy and vitality."

Many women would love to restore their libido but are ashamed or embarrassed to admit it and seek help and yet, in my medical practice, the vast majority of women who want their libido back are successful at reigniting it. A healthy sex drive comes with a kind of "sashay," or mojo, that signals confidence and self-esteem, that aura of having a special secret and a Cheshire Cat smile.

The goal of this book is to give women the knowledge and tools to restore libido and recreate a satisfying sex life.

Prioritizing Your Own Health

Are you ready to embark on a journey back into your own body and back into the arms of your partner? Are you ready for joy, pleasure, and energetic good health, including healthy sexuality? If this direction feels right to you, it's time to give some thought to where you fall on your own list of priorities.

With patient after patient in my practice, I've seen how women fall to the bottom of their own priority lists. Rejuvenating libido is a multidimensional process. Be prepared to invest time, attention, and energy in this journey. Be prepared for a change in diet, a shift in physical activity patterns, and a new awareness of where time and energy are best spent.

After prime reproductive age, libido works best when it is tended and cultivated. A lot of my patients come in well-informed but are still surprised when I explain that no magic pills will bring their sexy back. "Really? I have to give up fast food?" they'll ask, right after telling me how much they would like lose weight and stop taking high blood pressure medications.

The benefits of sex

The benefits of keeping the sexual fires burning are numerous. Here are a few good reasons to restore a lost libido. Each will be explored in detail in later chapters:

- Sex is a good cardiovascular workout.
- Sex helps maintain flexibility and strength.
- Sex relieves stress.
- Sex increases levels of important feel-good brain chemicals and hormones.
- Sex helps partners bond and create greater intimacy.
- Sex improves sleep quality.
- Sex helps protect men against prostate cancer.

For some women, low libido is a normal part of the aging process, but for others it's a telltale warning sign of less-than-optimal health. When a woman is physically unwell, her libido is one of the first things to go. My approach to helping any woman with hormone balance-related issues combines hormone-balancing therapies with a broad range of other interventions that improve libido and overall health.

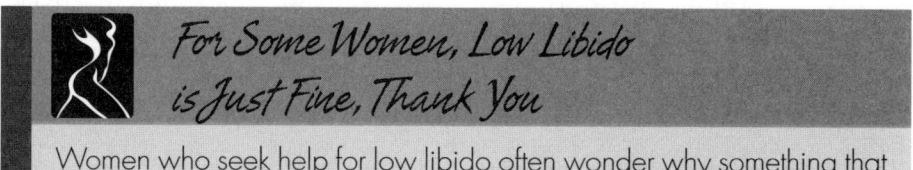

For Some Women, Low Libido is Just Fine, Thank You

Women who seek help for low libido often wonder why something that dominated their younger lives has dimmed or vanished altogether. They miss those intense feelings and the satisfaction of sexual connection.

This being said, not all women consider a drop in libido as a problem to be solved. Women of any age may choose not to resurrect a libido that has gone south. Some might never have had a strong interest in sex or a strong drive toward it. Although they might, in response to perimenopausal (just before menopause) or menopausal symptoms, seek out the help of a physician like me who aids in hormone balancing, they aren't there to locate a lost libido.

Many women, especially after menopause, are satisfied with a sex life that's in neutral. They may be relieved to be free of those youthful primal urges and want to devote their attention and energy to other creative aspects of life. Don't let anyone tell you that you *should* turn a flagging libido around if it's not something that is important to *you*.

Bioidentical Hormones, Properly Prescribed

Surveys show that menopausal women are the most likely to have low libido, which makes sense because menopause brings a significant drop in levels of the very hormones that help create sex drive. Women who have had surgery to remove their ovaries are plunged into instant menopause and have the most pronounced and sudden loss of desire for sex. Low hormones are the physical reality behind many lost libidos.

If you have been scared away from hormone replacement therapy (HRT) by warnings that it causes cancers, strokes and heart disease, I would like to reassure you now that hormones *can* be replaced safely and effectively when they are *bioidentical.* Bioidentical hormones are carbon copies of the hormones made by the human body.

Many doctors, even some who use bioidentical hormones, believe that restoring libido in a woman is simply a matter of giving her a prescription for testosterone. In Chapter 5 you'll find out why this magic bullet approach can backfire and cause more problems than it solves. Optimal health and libido is created by hormone *balance.*

If your hormones are out of balance, restoring sex drive will usually include hormone replacement. I intend, in this book, to demystify hormone replacement and give you science-based reassurance about the safety of properly prescribed bioidentical hormones.

But there's more to it than hormones

Patients with low libido often arrive in my office with the hope that I'll be able to prescribe a magic pill to bring it back. They've heard that I specialize in bioidentical hormone replacement and are looking for a combination of hormones that will transport them back to their sexier days.

Libido certainly does have a lot to do with the balance, or imbalance, of certain hormones, and I routinely test women's hormone levels. Based on what testing and symptoms tell us, I will usually prescribe bioidentical hormones as part of a treatment plan.

However, although bioidentical hormones can make a big difference in restoring libido, they're only part of the big picture. Here are some of the physical factors that can derail libido even when hormones are balanced:

- High levels of stress hormones.
- Lack of exercise.
- Poor diet, most often too much sugar and refined carbohydrates.
- Medications or recreational drugs that reduce libido.
- Excess alcohol.

I'll discuss these non-hormonal sex sinkers and others in detail in later chapters.

Your Man and Your Libido

Men can have their own issues with libido and sexuality that contribute to or worsen the issues their partners face. Some men experience the stereotypical "midlife crisis," which can contribute to marital turmoil that makes one or both partners avoid sex. Other men start to settle into what might be appropriately termed a midlife decline, which may include loss of energy, loss of libido, or erection problems that lead to avoidance of sex. It is amazing to me how many couples have not discussed their lack of sex and intimacy with their partners. Many women are afraid they will insult their spouse if they mention his erection issues, but men can be also be successfully treated for low libido and erectile dysfunction (ED).

Some men aren't interested in making sex an enjoyable experience for their partner. It's no surprise that a woman whose sex life has been unsatisfying loses her desire for sex. And lastly, some men (and to be fair, some women) let themselves go so much that they are no longer sexually appealing to their partners. Libido can be chilled by either partner's obesity, sloppiness, or complacency, especially in a long-term union.

The Psychology of Libido

We've established that libido is tied to physical factors, but for women in particular, it's also strongly tied to emotions, self-esteem, trust and other psychological factors. We all know the saying about the brain being the most important sex organ. Most women need to feel loved, loving and secure to be in the mood for sex; desire grows most reliably when relationships are on firm ground and self-esteem is intact. Brain chemicals that control mood, intertwined with thoughts and emotions, can affect the way women think and feel about everything, including sex.

An approach to restoring libido that addresses the whole instead of its individual working parts has the best chance of success. A woman's lifestyle choices play a pivotal role. Does she live a harried, stressed-out life? Does she eat poorly? Does she exercise? Does she take care of herself or devote herself completely to others? Is she making choices in her life that are pushing her physically and psychologically into a state of poor health? A body and mind in poor health won't readily enter the psychological and physical states necessary for pleasurable sex.

Pain during intercourse is a common reason women lose interest in sex. Painful sex is often the result of hormonal changes that thin the walls of the vagina and reduce natural lubrication, but it can also spring from a history of sexual abuse or sexual difficulties. The body can create physical pain where there is unresolved psychological pain. If past or present trauma underlies pain related to sex, it needs to be addressed before libido can be restored.

Studies have shown that some women have normal physical responses to sexual arousal yet they have no desire for sex. For example, their sexual organs may respond to an erotic film, but that response doesn't necessarily reach the brain and translate into wanting to have sex. For these women, there is a disconnect between the body's physical response and the level of desire perceived by the mind. Relationship problems may be to blame, or the overwhelming stress of day-to-day life may have literally shut down the connections between the mind, emotions and body.

Barbara Carrellas, who wrote the excellent book, *Urban Tantra* (Celestial Arts 2007) says, "The statement 'I don't have time for sex' usually has little to do with time or sex. More often, it means 'I'm tired,' or 'I really need to work,' or 'I'd really *rather* work.' It can mean 'I want to spend more time with the children' or 'I have spent way, way too much time with the children.' It often means 'I need some time completely to myself—away from everything and everyone. I have nothing left to give.' Our desire for sex (especially for partner sex) can be depleted by, among other things, anxiety, depression, antidepressants, lack of work, overwork, or even just an obsession with our children. It's not that we don't have the time for sex, it's just that other things seem more important, necessary, or enjoyable than sex. Ironically, sex is probably just the thing to alleviate the depression, exhaustion, anxiety, and obsession..."

Mindfulness: The secret ingredient

I do have one secret ingredient in my libido restoration recipe, and that is *mindfulness*. It's the last thing my patients expect their physician to bring up, but this particular state of mind can be enormously supportive of a healthy libido.

Many a woman tells me about her mind wandering during sex, to the chores of daily life and the never-ending to-do lists. These intruding thoughts keep her from fully engaging and enjoying the sensual experience that she is having. Without engagement of the brain, adequate arousal may not happen, and this will usually result in a less than satisfying sexual experience.

Mindfulness is about being in the moment, about finding ways to be present and aware, still the mind's chatter and fully engage the sensory, sensual self. When coupled with a healthy body that has hormone levels conducive to good libido, mindfulness will take your sex life—and your relationship with your partner—to a level it may never have reached before. As with the other aspects of my advice for improving libido, practicing mindfulness will benefit much more than your sex life.

A New Consciousness of Libido

As libido ebbs with age, and the day-to-day humdrum and stresses of life threaten to douse romantic fires altogether, we have the opportunity to transform sex into a source of pleasure and deep connectedness with our partner, as well as a self-healing, self-loving practice that isn't dictated by the drive to repopulate the planet. Sexuality in midlife shifts from an intense biological imperative to a conscious choice.

In making an intentional choice to rejuvenate libido, we also choose to embrace life and its pleasures fully. While transforming a flagging libido can be as simple as taking the right hormones, it's more often a multilayered process involving commitment, time and energy. The rewards are well worth it.

You already know my story, and I can tell you that my choice to devote attention and effort toward rebuilding an intimate connection with my husband has benefits that go well beyond our sex lives. It has made our marriage stronger and allowed us to explore new facets of our partnership.

Every day in my medical practice, I meet women just like you and I who have a similar choice. I also see many variations on the theme of lost libido, and it's important to understand that everyone expresses their sexuality, or lack of it, a little bit differently. There is no single definition of healthy libido. Part of the journey to restoring libido is to rediscover and recreate your concept of a healthy, happy, satisfying sex life. Your libido is unique, and your plan for restoring it—or for making it stronger and better than it's ever been—will be unique as well.

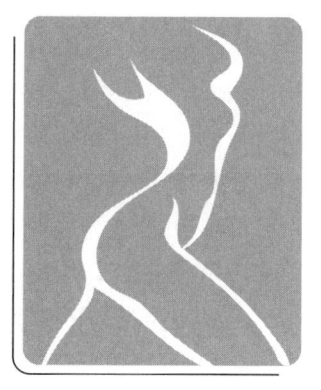

CHAPTER 2

What is Sexy?

At 55, Sally was convinced that her sex life was over. She had loved sex in her younger years, but it had become unpleasant at best and painful at worst. Her husband still wanted to be sexual with her, though, and she was carrying around a lot of anger and hostility about his continuing advances. Sally's resistance made her avoid any kind of cuddling or physical closeness with her husband. "I can't wait for him to lose his libido," she told me at our first appointment, "so we can be on the same track. I think it's time for all that to be done with. Isn't it natural for me to stop wanting sex as soon as I can't get pregnant anymore?"

If you've experienced a loss of libido, you might have entertained thoughts similar to Sally's. "Now that my reproductive years are over, why should I even *have* a libido? Doesn't sex drive come from the instinct to procreate and pass on our genes?"

The answer to these questions is yes and no. Yes, it's true that sex drive does naturally fade in many women as they age and their hormones change. And no, aging does not have to mean the end of one's sex life. Far from it!

Wanting sex is about more than hormones. The desire for sex, especially in women, can be complicated. Over the centuries, many a sex researcher from Hippocrates on has thrown in the towel when it comes to figuring out what makes women tick sexually. Sex surveys of women, particularly those over the age of 40, are notorious for returning mixed results. Woven into the complicated puzzle of individual libido we have biology, biochemistry, culture, religion, upbringing, health status, lifestyle, and the history and dynamics of current relationships that range from internet dating to decades of marriage. The process of restoring a lost libido is unique to each and every woman.

Feeling sexy is an integral part of wanting to have sex, but what is sexy?

Youth is Sexy

Sex is Mother Nature's way of ensuring that the human species continues, and from mid-puberty through the 20s, the sex drives are at their peak. For women, youth is, and always has been, equated with the sexual ideal. There are good reasons for this. From an evolutionary point of view, a man has a better chance of passing on his genes with a young, healthy woman. Biologically speaking, a younger woman is more likely to get pregnant and bear a healthy child. Men are hardwired to desire youthful sexiness.

In industrialized cultures the youthful, sexy woman is used to promote and market literally everything and anything, but most of all it's used to sell the illusion that youthful sexiness can be achieved with clothing, cosmetics, miracle potions, lotions and supplements, hair coloring, plastic surgery, exercise machines, diets and the like. Photos of models and celebrities are intensely Photoshopped to make us believe they are magically decades younger. (This illusion is contradicted by raw tabloid pictures of celebrities without makeup, complete with wrinkles, baggy eyes, cellulite and stretch marks—one of the few ways tabloids help more than they hurt.) Senior celebrities make public appearances with eerily smooth, masklike faces that have had all expression stretched out of them, and somehow they believe that we will believe they are younger than their actual age and thus more desirable.

Everywhere, and from the cradle to the grave, women are bombarded with the message that unless they look like they're 20-something, they're not sexually desirable. While biologically speaking this has a thread of truth, the beauty of being human is that we have the mental, emotional and physical means to move past our biology and our less-than-perfect bodies to create a deeply satisfying sex life at any age.

Cultural Sexiness is Ever-Changing

What's sexy at any given moment in human history, anywhere around the globe, has some consistent biological imperatives, but culturally what's sexy is constantly changing. The ever-shifting sands of sexiness have spawned volumes of literature and creativity, from Egyptian murals and medical textbooks to romance novels and porn, as well as entire branches of academia, endless movies and a multi-billion dollar beauty and anti-aging industry.

The ways in which humans act out their sexuality are profoundly affected by what their cultures consider sexy—and what they consider taboo. Cultural beliefs about sex can become so ingrained that they're not even perceived as negotiable… that is until the next generation changes them.

While watching TV might cause you to believe that, sexually speaking, we live in an incredibly permissive era, Dr. Laura Berman, author of *real sex for real women: intimacy, pleasure & sexual wellbeing* (DK Adult 2008) says otherwise: "Even though sex is used to sell everything from chocolate and ice cream to cars and aftershave, we are less likely than the previous generation to be adventurous or sexually self-accepting... Challenge any view that confines your sexuality and begin to fully understand your sexual desires and needs. Our sexuality is as fluid and diverse as the cultures on the Earth—an ever-evolving sexual continuum."

A Short History of Sex

It's worthwhile to take a quick look back at sexual attitudes and practices through history, simply to remind ourselves how often and dramatically the cultural rules of sex morph into new paradigms.

Relics, cave paintings and human remains from the time of the earliest humans suggest that 300,000 years ago, at least some of our ancestors had varied and recreational sex lives that included sex with more than one partner, same-sex partners, cross-dressing, and sex for physical fitness and spiritual enrichment. There's even evidence that prehistoric humans engaged in group sex and bondage and used sex toys.

Ancient Egyptians were liberal in their attitudes toward sex. Although it's difficult to make sweeping statements about a civilization that lasted 3,000 years, it's probably safe to generalize that ancient Egyptians, who believed in gods and goddesses, also believed that both men and women were entitled to active sex lives. Sex was both sacred and an important part of everyday life. Incest was common among the ruling classes.

In ancient Greece, it was considered normal for grown men in the upper classes to have wives, mistresses, *and* teenaged male lovers. Wives were treated with respect but weren't considered appropriate targets for male sexual passion; that was reserved for boys and mistresses. Prostitution was illegal.

During most of the nearly 500 years of the Roman Empire, it was acceptable for men to have sex with other men, but unacceptable (and for certain periods illegal) for a married woman to have sex with anyone but her husband.

Many of the ancient Hebrews had multiple wives but with strict rules governing property ownership and inheritance. With the advent of Christianity, some interpretations of the Bible led to the conclusion that sex for any purpose besides procreation was sinful, which led to the practice of men having sex with their wives only for procreation, and secretly having recreational sex with mistresses, slaves and servants.

For thousands of years of Chinese history, it was standard practice in the upper classes for men to have a hierarchy of multiple wives, or a wife and multiple concubines.

Marriage and the nuclear family as we know it today is a fairly recent phenomenon. For most of human history, marriage was a financial and political arrangement made by parents. Sex was part of marriage, but for men, also took place outside of marriage. Within marriage, women had few if any legal rights and were traded, bought and sold as property. In many cultures, men were free to rape, beat and even kill their wives, without consequence—and still are in some developing countries. These types of arrangements typically did not lead to a rewarding sex life for women!

In Europe, the Christian religion wasn't part of marriage until the 1500s, and the concept of romance in marriage came much later.

Today in France, although not legally sanctioned, having sex outside of marriage is widely accepted. In Italy, even with the Catholic church in charge of sexuality, it is common for a man to have a mistress, but the practice is legally and publicly condemned.

In America, women did not even have the right to vote until 1920, so it's fair to say that American women's lives have been dramatically transformed over the past century, from sexual oppression and repression, to the 60s era of birth control and sex, drugs and rock 'n roll, to financial independence and unparalleled personal, political and sexual freedom. Given centuries of oppression compared to a mere few decades of freedom, it's no wonder women are in need of a new sexual paradigm. And yet, according to an *American Economic Journal* article, "The Paradox of Declining Female Happiness," women are less happy now than at any time in the past 40 years, primarily because of high levels of fatigue and stress caused by working outside the home while also maintaining the primary "emotional responsibility" for home and family.

Sexy Body Types

Culture dictates what body type is considered sexy. Just 200 years ago the ideal woman was round and voluptuous—overweight in comparison to modern fashion models and movie stars. Back then, ample proportions were a symbol of wealth and health. In fact, for much of human history, thin women have not been considered sexy. Even the sex symbols of 1940s and 50s America would be considered voluptuous by today's standards.

Two hundred years ago being tan meant you were a poor person who had to work outdoors in the sun—it was not sexy. Being pasty white was sexy, so much so that even men covered their faces with white powder. In the 1960s and 70s being tan meant you were wealthy enough to have leisure time and vacation in tropical locales—it was the height of fashion and sexiness.

For much of the 1800s in Europe and America, large busts and tiny waists were the prevailing fashion trend. Victorian women were considered sexually "loose" if they dared show a bare ankle or had more than a sip of alcohol… but showing cleavage was acceptable, especially if it was garnished with lace. By the roaring twenties women were slugging back gin and wearing skirts above the knee.

In the 1960s the birth control pill ushered in a new era of sex for women, in which they were free to have sex without fear of becoming pregnant. Then the rise of HIV/AIDs brought more caution to sexual liaisons.

Sex and religion

Throughout human history, religion has often been responsible for dictating women's roles and "appropriate" sexuality. In cultures where women's power and sexuality are embraced as positives, female sexuality has tended to find a more healthy expression. In male-dominated cultures where women are suppressed or considered to be the property of men, the extreme opposite has been true.

Although Islam has been one of the most consistently repressive religions regarding women and their sexuality, celibacy is not recommended for men. Sex is forbidden outside of marriage (although in practice infidelity among men is common), and sex within marriage is a religious duty for both husband and wife. And yet, the Muslim countries of the Middle East brought us belly dancing, which was traditionally supposed to be done within the harem in front of women only. (Highly doubtful, as men would not want to miss out on that particular art form.)

Likewise, women in India are highly repressed and yet it was Buddhist India that brought us the Kama Sutra, the ultimate guide to love, sex and every imaginable position in which to have sex. Hindu India brought us Tantric sex, which will be mentioned in more detail in later chapters.

Medicine dictates sexiness

As Christian religions became ever more-involved in the sex lives of their followers in Europe and America, medical doctors jumped right onto the "women who enjoy sex are sinful" bandwagon. Trusted American 19th-century medical "experts" such as John Harvey Kellogg and Harvard's Edward H. Clarke, M.D., maintained that women who enjoyed sex were sick or improper. Women accused of being too sexual might be condemned to barbaric medical procedures or a stay in a mental institution. It was considered a medical fact that sex after menopause made a woman ill. Victorian doctors manually masturbated women to relieve hysteria, seemingly unaware that the moans and muscle spasms being elicited were orgasms.

In the 1940s, sex researchers began to clear some of the confusion about sexuality through the use of scientific research. Scientists such as Alfred Kinsey began to demystify the physical side of sex and to make it an acceptable topic of conversation in relationships and in the culture in general. But even this dispassionate, seemingly objective way of looking at sex was impacted by culture.

In the 1960s, William Masters and Elizabeth E. Johnson, the pioneering authors of *The Human Sexual Response*, described sex in four stages: *excitement*, where the body shifts into an aroused state; *plateau*, or intense arousal that has not yet peaked in orgasm; *orgasm*; and then a *resolution* phase. Desire was assumed to come first, before these four steps kicked in. This idea of the progression of sexual arousal through orgasm took hold in our culture as the "correct" progression—the progression to be expected and aimed for in most sexual encounters. Any variation on this theme of four-stage heterosexual intercourse came to be seen as abnormal.

Modern guidelines used to diagnose sexual dysfunction and low libido are also based on the Masters and Johnson model. Based on her experience as a clinical sex therapist and counselor, Gina Ogden, Ph.D., began to think that the high numbers of women who supposedly had low libido didn't actually have a problem—they just didn't equate a good sexual experience with the kind of sex they *thought* they were supposed to be having. Dr. Ogden created the ISIS (Integrating Spirituality in Sexuality) survey, and more than 3,800 women and men responded. Amazingly, less than one percent of the women who participated in this national survey said that intercourse was required for them to have a satisfactory sexual experience!

Where Masters and Johnson saw sexual arousal as a linear progression toward orgasm, researchers like Dr. Rosemary Basson of the University of British Columbia argued in 1999 that women, at least, operate in a more circular pattern. Desire can precede stimulation or be triggered by it. Satisfaction is possible at any of the stages. And orgasm isn't necessarily the ultimate goal.

The idea that sex is always supposed to go from desire to arousal to intercourse to orgasm to cuddling and sleep is a culturally prescribed idea, just like the idea that 20-somethings and 30-somethings are the only people who should be having sex.

A New Paradigm

For most female animals, mating is tolerated in response to prodding from hormones and instincts and is an emotionally unmoving event that is over in a matter of seconds. Humans are among the few species that have sex for fun. We can desire and enjoy sex any time, whether we're fertile or not—because human libido isn't dictated by fertility (although women can feel more impulsive and urgent about having sex during certain parts of their cycles). A woman's libido is tied to her hormones, but it's also woven into her thoughts, dreams, sensory experiences, creativity and feelings toward her partner.

Our current concepts of "normal" sexuality tend to be modeled on the sex drive and urgency of our reproductive years—having that surge of lust and following it with one or more bouts of potentially athletic, often orgasmic intercourse. But most of us will live a third or more of our lives after our prime reproductive years are over. Historically women past the age of 40 have had little opportunity or cultural context for cultivating a great sex life. We may, historically speaking, be creating a new paradigm right here and now.

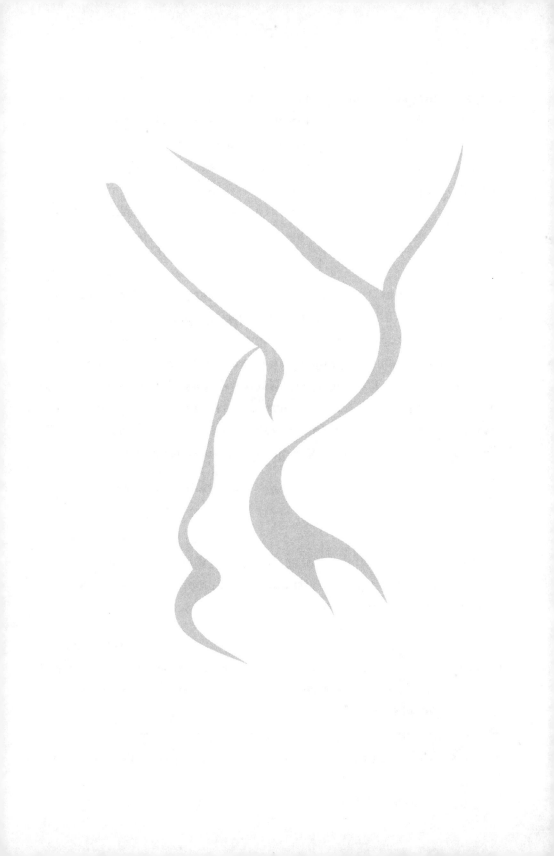

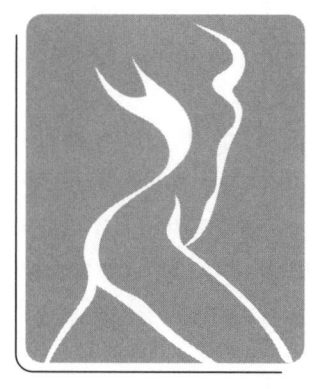

CHAPTER 3

Let's Get Physical – The Organs of Libido

So many of the concerns women bring to me can be boiled down to a single foundational question: "Am I normal?" Women want to know whether there's something *wrong* with them. This is no surprise, considering how often women encounter unrealistic images and ideas about how they're supposed to look and how they're supposed to respond to sexual cues or sexual stimulation.

For example, many women have breasts that are of obviously different sizes. I've even heard nicknames like "Mighty Righty" or "Hefty Lefty!" I reassure these women by telling them that asymmetry is absolutely normal—that actually, it's more the rule than the exception. Other women are concerned because their *labia minora*, the inner 'lips' that protect the opening of the vagina, are two different sizes. Or they think the labia minora are too long because they hang down past the edges of the *labia majora*, the outer lips. Surgical procedures that reduce the size of the labia minora are rising in popularity, and so are injections that 'plump' the labia minora in postmenopausal women. I don't recommend these kinds of procedures because nerves can be severed and sensation can be lost.

Female genitals, just like every other part of the female body, can vary a lot in size, shape and symmetry. They change through time, childbearing and menopause. All of these variations in appearance go hand in hand with variations in the ways women's bodies operate, feel, react and respond.

In this chapter, you'll get an in-depth tour of the female body—in particular, the parts of the body that participate in generating libido and pleasure with sex. As you move through this user's manual for your organs of libido in midlife and beyond, you'll see how dramatically different the bodies of women can be while still falling into the category of "normal." The organs of libido are affected by childbirth, hysterectomy and the aging process, particularly during the shift into menopause.

Touch, sight, hearing and smell create and maintain libido just as much—if not more than—the genitals or other parts of the body typically considered to be erotic, especially for women.

Huge variations exist in the ways that women get interested and aroused, and in the ways they get pleasure from sex. Because these differences go back to the brain, the most important sexual organ, I'll start with a look at the senses. Through your eyes, ears, skin and nose, you absorb cues that powerfully impact libido.

The Sounds, Smells, Sights and Sensations of Desire

Birdsong, cricket song, mating displays, the scent of a fertile female animal carried on the wind to a ready and willing male, the touch of a man's hand on the small of a woman's back: these are all messages between males and females that create the urge to merge. Every animal that needs a mate to reproduce needs to be able to send and receive signals through smells, sounds, touch or physical changes in order to mate at the right times. Most animals only use one or two of these mechanisms, but humans can send and receive all of these types of signals.

When medical experts talk about restoring libido, the sensory organs don't get talked about nearly as much as the vagina, vulva, clitoris and other erogenous zones like the breasts and the buttocks, but they're every bit as important. In youth, we send and receive those sensory signals without really being aware of them or recognizing their power over us. As the spontaneous desire and arousal of youth give way to a more conscious approach to being sexual, the senses come to play a bigger role in libido.

Chemical 'signals' about fertility and desire—sometimes referred to as *pheromones*—are sent out and sensed by the opposite sex. Touch both attracts and arouses. Your sense of sight can turn you on when you watch a great sex scene in a romantic movie or your mate undresses in front of you. Women can use their imagination, fantasy or erotica to become turned on, some even to the point of orgasm. They can imagine sensory details so vividly that their bodies' sexual responses are triggered.

Touch connects, arouses and heals

Skin is the largest organ, and some have called it the largest sexual organ. Consistent touching and being touched are good reasons to keep sex going through midlife and beyond.

From the time you were a six-week-old fetus in your mother's belly, you had a sense of touch. Children who don't get adequate touch during infancy and childhood are at risk for slow development and poor health. In the early 20th century, before the importance of touch for a baby's growth was understood, nearly every baby sent to an orphanage failed to develop

41

normally or died. These babies were only touched when they were fed, and their bodies simply shut down.

We don't lose our need for touch in adulthood. When we're touched regularly, we feel loved, calmed and accepted. It's a kind of sensory nutrition that everyone needs.

Oxytocin, the cuddle and bonding hormone

A hormone called *oxytocin* is produced in both men and women in response to loving touch. Oxytocin is involved in the strong motherly feelings a woman has toward her baby, particularly during cuddling or nursing. Nipple stimulation directly raises oxytocin levels. Sometimes called the "bonding hormone" or the "cuddle hormone," oxytocin has soothing, calming effects on the body and balances the effects of stress hormones such as cortisol. Orgasm causes a strong release of oxytocin—that's what makes you want to cuddle afterward. It plays a role in creating feelings of love, bonding and trust between people.

The intensity of touch during sex is greater than in any other kind of touch. Full-body contact during sex usually involves lots of stroking, rubbing, bare skin on bare skin and kissing—and the surge in oxytocin levels is correspondingly higher than any you'd experience with a brief contact in passing or a long couch-cuddling session. By being sexual with your partner, you're giving yourself (and your partner) the gift of a surge in this nurturing, soothing hormone.

When oxytocin levels go up, testosterone and estrogen levels go up too. By having sex and engaging in other kinds of touch, you create a hormonal environment in your body that will then create the desire for more sex and more touch. Even lying together and touching (without clothing is best) can help jump-start desire by increasing oxytocin. It begins a cycle that propagates itself.

Sound, sight and sexuality

Just as people have different learning styles, they also have different sexual styles. Each person tends to favor one of the senses over the others. Some people are kinesthetic and so prefer to experience the world through touch; some are auditory and process information best by hearing, while others are visual learners who have to "see it to believe it." Where one person's sense of smell might be strongly woven into her sex drive, another person might be less olfactory and more visual, tactile or auditory.

If you're the kind of person who loves to listen to music, and whose moods can be affected by music and the spoken word; if you learn best through listening; if you can spend hours on the phone with a friend, then you are likely someone whose primary way of interpreting the world is through the sense of hearing. If you fit this description, chances are good that you'll get more out of a sexual experience if your partner talks to you while you're making love or if you listen to evocative music during your time together. If, on the other hand, you depend more on your eyes than on your ears for your experience of the world, you're probably more visual than auditory, and you're more likely to get a libido boost from looking at something that arouses you. There's no single right way to get turned on for either gender.

If partners don't understand and take into account these differences in making sense of the world, frustration and low libido can result. She wants him to come to bed freshly bathed and smelling great, so she puts fresh flowers next to the bed where she waits for him, dressed in a lavender-scented nightgown. He doesn't care how she smells—he just wants her to be naked and available, out in the open where he can see her every curve and crevice. Neither of these partners will be satisfied if they don't consider which senses are most associated with libido for them, and then have a conversation about what they want.

The Scent of Desire: Pheromones and Libido

Why do the menstrual cycles of women who live together tend to become synchronized? The consensus is that this is due to pheromones—chemicals made in the body that give off specific scents through skin, urine and sweat. We're not consciously aware of those scents, but they carry information that triggers hormonal changes strong enough to alter the timing of women's menstrual cycles. Scents can alter levels of libido-inducing hormones in men, too. *Copulins* are chemicals found in female vaginal secretions, and they're especially abundant during ovulation. When a man catches wind of these, his testosterone levels rise.

Animal musk, which is a part of many fragrances made for men and women, is considered to be a very sexy scent—not surprising, since it's rich in chemicals that are almost identical to human testosterone. In one experiment, women who sniffed musk every day for a period of time had shortened menstrual cycles and more frequent ovulation.

Research shows that women are wired to choose a mate whose immune system contains elements her own immune system lacks, which is apparently a physical trait that we can detect through our sense of smell. This was most vividly proven by an experiment involving T-shirts worn by various men. Women were asked to take a whiff of each shirt and tell researchers which they preferred. The T-shirts they chose turned out to be from men who were more genetically compatible with them—with whom they were more likely to produce a healthy child.

Despite the ads you might have seen for pheromone potions, no one has actually been able to isolate human pheromones yet; those found in perfumes and colognes come from animals or are manufactured in a laboratory. Still, every woman has scents that turn her on: a favorite cologne, maybe, or the aroma of her man's post-workout sweat.

Losing Your Sense of Smell

Anosmia, or the loss of the sense of smell, often causes a big drop in libido. Smells strongly evoke emotions and memories, so when this sense is lost, depression is a common result. Those who have lost their sense of smell may have to force themselves to eat. As we age, our sensitivity to smell declines, and this can play a role in low libido. In turn, I have had women tell me that a few months after starting hormone replacement therapy their sense of smell returned.

For women with an acute sense of smell, the wrong cologne or body odor can be a big turn-off, but the right odors can be an intense turn-on. Scents are powerful, and women with low libido might explore scents to promote sexy thoughts and physical arousal.

Non-Genital Zones of Pleasure

The word *erogenous* (pronounced *err-AHG-uh-nuss*) is made up of the Greek words for "love" (*eros*) and "produce" (*genein*). An erogenous zone is a part of the body that produces erotic feelings and sexual urges when touched. The genitals are erogenous zones, of course, but the breasts and anus deserve a mention here as well.

Just as the appearance of breasts can vary, so can their sensitivity as organs of libido. Some women love having their partners play with, suck on or caress their breasts and nipples. For others, nipple or breast stimulation feels so-so or even unpleasant. Both are normal. Imbalances in estrogen, progesterone and testosterone can affect the sensitivity of these areas.

The anus is also an erogenous zone. It has a very high concentration of nerve endings, and some people enjoy being stimulated in that area. Not everyone has an interest in going there—sometimes because of strong cultural taboos around anal sex and anal stimulation, sometimes because it just plain doesn't feel good. Any anal play should be preceded with a shower, a bath or some other way of getting the area completely clean. If you or your partner touches or penetrates the anus, that part should be washed with soap and water before it touches the vulva (exterior part of the female genitals) or enters the vagina.

As women age, the perineum, which is the area between anus and vagina, shrinks. Once this occurs, it's easier for bacteria to move from the anal area into the urethra and vagina, which can make women more susceptible to urinary tract and vaginal infections. Take extra care to keep these areas clean, and keep in mind that bioidentical hormone replacement may help counteract this shrinkage.

Other non-genital parts of the body might carry more of an erotic charge for you than the breasts or anus. Loving touch or kisses on the neck, feet, thighs, ankles, buttocks or the small of the back can be highly arousing. As you explore ways to heighten libido and enjoy sex, be aware of your own non-genital erogenous zones and encourage your partner to go there to help you get in the mood.

The Genital Zones

For most women the genitals are the primary zone of sexual pleasure, so it's important when restoring sex drive to be well-acquainted with the various parts, what can go wrong, and how to restore parts that aren't working.

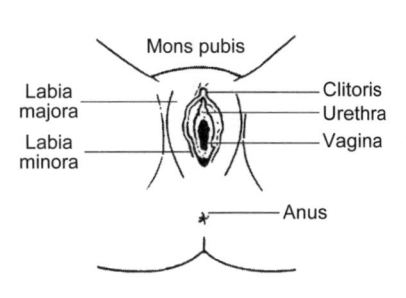

The vulva

First, let's get the terminology straight. Although the external parts of the female genitals—the outer and inner labia—are often referred to as the vagina, these parts are actually called the vulva. The vagina is the actual passageway that opens into the area of the vulva and extends up to the cervix, at the base of the uterus.

As I mentioned, one woman's external genitalia can be very different from another's. The *mons* (the small deposit of fat that sits over the pubic bone, above the clitoris) can be generously sized or smaller. Patterns of pubic hair growth and texture of hair differ a lot between women. Some women shave, wax or have laser therapy to remove much of their pubic hair; this is purely a matter of personal preference for the individual woman and her partner. Aging can cause pubic hair to thin.

Every fetus starts out female. A fetus with a male chromosome will eventually begin to produce more of the masculinizing hormones, and the tissues that would otherwise become female reproductive organs grow into male organs. A male fetus starts out with the raw materials for the fleshier outer lips of the vagina and the *labia majora*; and then, with the right hormone stimulation during the earliest stages of development, these parts develop into a scrotum, the sac that holds the testicles. The *labia minora* are the inner lips of the vagina that sit inside the labia majora. They are thinner than the labia majora and can vary greatly in size. In some women, the labia minora are narrow enough to sit hidden inside the outer labia; in others they can be up to two inches long from base to ends and hang well below the labia majora. Inside the labia minora, just next to the vaginal opening, are several *Bartholin's glands*, which produce fluids that help to lubricate the vulva and vagina during sex. During ovulation, the texture of these fluids becomes more alkaline, which helps sperm make their way through the vagina and up through the uterus to meet the egg.

Hormonal changes in midlife and beyond cause the labia to lose fullness and flexibility. In extreme cases, I've even seen a fusing of the inner and outer labia in older women. In those cases, a little estrogen and testosterone do wonders and allow the labia to gradually be separated from each other as they plump up.

At the place where the labia minora meet is one of the most talked-about female organs of libido: the clitoris.

The clitoris

Although at first glance, a penis and a clitoris seem about as different as night and day, they have a lot in common.

A penis and a clitoris are made up of the same tissues; in a male fetus, the bud of tissue that becomes the female clitoris becomes a penis. Most women don't know that the clitoris is about four inches long—the same length as the average non-erect penis. The clitoris has 'legs' called *crurae* that extend well into the vagina. The part of the clitoris that can be seen and touched outside of the vagina is the *glans*, which lies under a hood analogous to the foreskin of the penis. Although the average clitoral glans is about half the size of a pencil eraser, it can vary in size, and swells during arousal. With menopause and a drop in testosterone, the clitoris can become smaller and less sensitive and for some women, this makes it more difficult to have an orgasm. A small dose of bioidentical testosterone can help restore clitoral sensitivity.

Some women like to have the clitoris rubbed hard and fast or enjoy strong grinding. Others like a much lighter touch and find direct pressure to be overwhelming. Women's differing levels of sensitivity in the clitoris and vagina may have to do with differences in the number of nerve endings found in these areas and with hormone levels.

Anatomy of an Orgasm

A common question women ask me is whether they should be having more than one kind of orgasm. They say to me, "Yes, I can have a clitoral orgasm, but big deal—I can't have the other kind." The vaginal orgasm, which happens without clitoral stimulation, has been the subject of hot debate among sex experts for decades.

Research shows that 80 percent of orgasms involve some type of clitoral stimulation. Only about 30 percent of women report having vaginal orgasms, but now that we understand how far the clitoris extends into the vagina, there may turn out to be little difference between a clitoral and a vaginal orgasm. An orgasm is an orgasm! Some sexual positions can stimulate the clitoris during intercourse to help an orgasm occur during intercourse. Raising the woman's hips up on a pillow can allow her partner's pelvis to press against her clitoris with each thrust, for example.

There's a big range of sensation in the experience of orgasm. Sex expert Annie Sprinkle did extensive field research and describes seven different kinds of orgasm: *dream-gasms* (during sleep), *microgasms* (orgasms that don't require physical stimulation), vaginal orgasms (including G-spot orgasms), *breath/energy* orgasms (achieved through breathwork and meditations that move sexual energy around in the body), clitoral orgasms (small to humongous, short to long), *megagasm* (the kind that blows the roof off and seems like a mystical experience), and combinations of these. While it isn't likely that this seven-category model will ever enter the mainstream, I like that Sprinkle is defining such a broad range of experience in women's orgasms.

Regardless of what stimulates it, orgasm follows a predictable course. First, arousal causes the heartbeat to quicken and muscles to tighten. The genital area becomes engorged with blood and feels warm. Breasts and clitoris swell a little, nipples stand out, and a red flush can develop on the face, neck or upper chest. Just before orgasm, the clitoris retracts a little beneath its hood. Orgasm officially begins with strong muscle contractions inside the vagina and in the uterus. Contractions might also be felt in the anus. These wavelike contractions can last for four to 15 seconds. Muscle contractions throughout the body, along with rising heart rate and blood pressure, are often part of an orgasm. Some women "ejaculate" clear fluid during orgasm.

Some women can orgasm just from thinking about sex, while others require long periods of stimulation. Others find orgasm frustratingly impossible to achieve. The quality and quantity of orgasms a woman has during sex will shift with hormonal changes, the passage of time, and her willingness to communicate what she wants with her partner. Masturbation can help women discover how their partners can best help them achieve climax. Working with awareness during intercourse or masturbation helps enhance the experience and can make orgasms more powerful and satisfying. For women who find orgasms difficult to achieve, the best approach is to let go of goal orientation during sex. A pleasurable and satisfying experience can be had without an orgasm, and if you allow yourself to feel and enjoy the entire experience, you might not even miss having one.

The vagina

Behind the urethra, which carries urine out of the body from the bladder, is the opening of the vagina. The root of the word *vagina* is Latin for "sheath" or "scabbard."

On average, an unaroused woman's vagina is 2 ½ inches deep along the front wall and about 3 inches deep along the back wall. It lies at about a 45-degree angle relative to the uterus. During arousal, the cervix moves up and the vagina becomes deeper and wider. It can be 4 or more inches deep when a woman reaches full arousal. Hard, pounding sex can hurt before you're fully aroused because your cervix has not yet moved up to make more room.

As any menopausal woman knows, the vagina changes dramatically when periods stop and hormone levels drop. Without the effects of estrogen, the tissues of the vagina become thinner and drier. The tissues may get so delicate that sex becomes painful.

Most women have heard about menopausal hot flashes and mood swings, but may be surprised by the vaginal dryness and shrinking that accompanies low hormone levels. I recently saw a menopausal patient who told me, "You know, I expected a lot of this. I expected my periods to stop. I expected hot flashes, night sweats and brain fog. But I did *not* expect my vagina to shrivel up." If sex is attempted when the vagina is in this condition, it can be very painful and even lead to vaginal muscle spasms. With proper hormone therapy and slow and careful stretching of the vagina, even a woman with extreme vaginal dryness and shrinking can get back to an active and pleasurable sex life.

It's wise to keep a water-based lubricant on hand for those times when the vagina isn't lubricated enough. Regular sex can help to maintain more blood flow to the vaginal walls.

Burning, itching, lack of lubrication and more frequent vaginal infections aren't uncommon from the mid-40s on. With changes in vaginal lubrication also come changes in pH, the acid-base balance of the vagina. This shift can lead to more frequent yeast infections, bacterial infections or vaginal discharge. Bioidentical hormones can help to restore better pH balance, and eating the way I recommend in Chapter 9 and taking my recommended supplements can also promote a whole-body state of balance that helps prevent infection.

Premenopausal women who feel that their vaginas are too loose as a result of childbirth are having so-called "vaginal rejuvenation surgeries" to tighten themselves up. I strongly discourage these surgeries! They can change sensation by severing nerves, and there is no guarantee that it will work. If you're close to menopause, your vagina is going to shrink soon enough, perhaps more than is comfortable. If you are premenopausal and concerned about your vaginal muscle tone, learn to do Kegel exercises. *More about Kegel exercises in Chapter 10.*

Prolapse Prevention

Another reason to keep your sex life alive: regular sex helps to strengthen the muscles that hold the uterus, vagina and bladder in place. Weakening and collapse of these structures is more common in women who have had a lot of babies, but hysterectomy and hormonal shifts in menopause can also predispose women to prolapse of the vagina or bladder. The vagina or uterus can literally fall and, in rare instances, can come completely out of the body. Symptoms of prolapse include feelings of pressure and difficulty with urination and defecation, but the early stages of prolapse do not always cause symptoms.

About 10 percent of women who have a hysterectomy develop a specific kind of prolapse called vaginal vault prolapse, where the top of the vagina begins to fall toward the opening of the vagina, and the vaginal walls weaken. If left to its own devices, the vagina may eventually turn itself inside out. Embarrassment often stands in the way of women who need medical help to reverse prolapse.

Hormone replacement can help prevent prolapse of the vagina, bladder and uterus, but some women will also require surgery to shore up the ligaments and other tissues that support the lower pelvic organs.

Thirty to 40 percent of women experience some degree of prolapse, usually after the age of 40, and most often after menopause.

The urethra

The urethra is the tube that carries urine out of the body. Its opening is just above the vaginal opening. As women age they become more susceptible to urinary tract problems, including infections, incontinence and urgency. Urinary tract infections cause inflammation in the urethra, which can make it painful to urinate. They can also cause urinary urgency, which is the feeling of needing to urinate, even though there may not be any urine in the bladder.

Urinary incontinence, which is very common in menopausal women, is an involuntary leakage of urine, especially when laughing or sneezing.

Although some urinary tract issues are a result of childbirth, which can stretch out and weaken supportive ligaments and other tissues, the urethra and bladder are affected by decreasing estrogen. The majority of urinary tract issues that I see respond very well to either estradiol, estriol (estrogens), testosterone or a combination, which can be applied to the vaginal/urethral area in a cream.

One patient came to see me with complaints of vaginal stenosis (a 'shrinkage' of the vagina) and severe vaginal dryness. She also had urge incontinence (inability to hold in her urine when her urge to go was strong) and stress incontinence (release of urine during sneezing or laughter). A surgery to shore up her bladder and improve her urinary control was already scheduled, but I asked her to hold off and see how she felt once she'd started bioidentical hormone therapy. After three months on bioidentical hormones, she came back to say that she no longer planned on having the surgery—she had no more urinary problems. This patient also shared that when she first started using the hormones she could barely get the vaginal applicator (used to administer some bioidentical hormones) into her vagina, but that it had since become very easy to slide in. "I forgot what I looked like down there before, but now that things are plumping up and it's back the way it used to be, I'm starting to remember!" she told me happily.

The G-spot: Fact or fiction?

In the 1950s, a researcher named Ernst Grafenberg suggested that an area just inside the front wall of the vagina seemed to be especially sensitive to sexual stimulation. Stimulating this area could lead to powerful orgasms or even to the release of female ejaculate. This spot was named the "G-spot" and many a woman has gone hunting for it since that time. While many have found their G-spot and enjoyed it a great deal, others keep coming up empty. Some research indicates that the G-spot exists, while other research discounts the existence of any such spot and attributes success in finding it to the power of belief. A survey of about 1,800 women concluded that 56 percent have a G-spot.

Medicine's best guess about the G-spot is that it isn't an actual physiologic structure, separate from the vagina and the clitoris. Some believe that it's the extension of the clitoris, but the more likely story is that the G-spot is actually the female prostate gland.

The area of the G-spot contains a kind of tissue called the *urethral sponge*, which strongly resembles the tissues that make up the male prostate gland. This tissue even manufactures prostate-specific antigen, the substance measured with the PSA test to check for prostate cancer. The urethral sponge is dotted with glands called *Skene's glands*, which seem to be the source of the female ejaculate that occasionally occurs in women during orgasm.

During arousal, the urethral sponge swells up much like the male penis. The same enzyme that creates male erection can be found in the urethral sponge. Women who have thicker tissues in the G-spot area are more likely to report having vaginal orgasms.

The best way to know whether you have a G-spot is to go looking for it. It helps to do so with a partner because the area can be hard to reach yourself—but plenty of toys designed for G-spot self-stimulation are available if you prefer to try to find it on your own. It's located from one to three inches up the front wall of the vagina. A hooked finger should be just about the right length for contacting it and pressing upward toward the belly button. The G-spot feels a bit like the roof of the mouth and might bulge out a little. Pressing into it or massaging it may make you feel as though you have to pee at first because this part of the vagina is close to the urethra. Continuing through this initial feeling can bring on intense orgasms in some women. When exploring the G-spot with a partner, it sometimes helps when he uses his other hand to put pressure on top of the pubic bone, so that the fingers are, in effect, meeting on the inside and outside.

About 40 percent of women sometimes experience ejaculation. The urethral sponge wraps around the urethra, and it becomes engorged during sexual arousal. During orgasm, the Skene's glands can eject a clear fluid that then emerges through the urethra.

The cervix

At the top of the vagina sits the cervix, the entryway to the uterus. A healthy cervix is pink, shiny and smooth. Cervical mucus helps to lubricate the vagina, and less is produced as menopause approaches. In menstruating women, the quality and quantity of cervical mucus changes over the course of the month; it can become almost like egg white during ovulation. Women can gauge their fertility by taking some cervical mucus between finger and thumb and stretching it apart. If it's stringy and wet, ovulation is probably occurring.

The cervix is its own sexual organ, which is why some OB/GYNs try to preserve it when doing a hysterectomy. Some women enjoy vigorous pounding on the cervix during sex. Its sensitivity varies across the menstrual cycle—during ovulation, the cervix can become tender. Deep penetration that hits the cervix can also cause soreness in the ovary that's producing the egg. Cervical sensitivity can be increased following procedures such as the cone biopsy used to remove pre-cancerous areas following a positive Pap test.

Be sure to get your Pap tests as recommended by your doctor to rule out cervical cancer. This test is safe and has brought the cure rate of cervical cancer up to more than 90 percent. Cervical cancer used to be a leading cause of cancer death in women, but the Pap test has led to a decline of 74 percent in deaths from this disease. Rates of cervical cancer death continue to fall each year. As cervical cancer tends to occur in midlife—between the ages of 20 and 50—you may not require yearly screening after menopause. After menopause, positive Paps can be caused by cervical atrophy; work with your doctor to make sure you avoid having unnecessary procedures to remove tissues that aren't really a risk.

Cervical polyps, or small non-cancerous tumors, are common in peri-menopausal women. These can cause bleeding between periods but can be easily taken care of by your OB/GYN if necessary

The uterus

This small, muscular organ plays a role in sexual pleasure when it contracts during orgasm. However, when things go wrong with the uterus, sexual desire and enjoyment can be affected.

One in four women has uterine fibroids at some point before menopause, and these can cause heavy bleeding or pain with intercourse. If used when fibroids are still small, a low dose of bioidentical progesterone can help women with fibroids. Once fibroids reach a certain critical mass, they start making their own hormones, and progesterone or any other hormone can stimulate their growth. Although many women are advised to have a hysterectomy for troublesome fibroids, this is rarely necessary. Minimally invasive procedures such as laparoscopy can remove even large fibroids without removal of the uterus. At menopause, fibroids virtually always shrink to the point where they are no longer an issue.

Many women have a "tipped" uterus. The uterus can be tipped forward or back, and both are normal. In women who have had endometriosis, scarring can be a cause of uterine tipping, but if there is no pain or other symptoms, a tipped uterus is nothing to worry about. One variation—the *retroverted* uterus, which is tipped backwards, so that the angle of uterus to vagina is decreased—can cause pain during sex, because the ovaries and uterus can be hit too hard by the man's penis. Women who feel a lot of pain during deep penetration, especially when in the female-superior position, may have this form of uterine tipping. Certain sexual positions will work better for women who have pain because of a tipped uterus; experimentation is the best way to figure out what's best. If there is no pain or other symptoms, but your doctor has told you that you have a tipped uterus, don't worry—it's normal. About 30 percent of women have a uterus that is tipped one way or the other.

Hysterectomy

Some of the most miserable patients I see are women who have had a hysterectomy, but they are also the ones who respond most quickly and dramatically to hormone replacement.

Hysterectomy—the removal of the uterus—causes a drop in all of the sex hormones. If the ovaries are also removed, the result is instant surgical menopause. Some women wake up from surgery with hot flashes. Even if the ovaries are spared, their blood supply is compromised by hysterectomy, and they will usually stop producing hormones altogether within two years.

I can't stress enough that women should consider every other option carefully before getting a hysterectomy. Many doctors will "sell" their patients on a hysterectomy by insisting that "all your problems will be over once it's out," but I can tell you that nothing is further from the truth. As the late Dr. John Lee, author of the classic book *What Your Doctor May Not Tell You about Menopause* (co-written with Virginia Hopkins) used to say, "Hysterectomy is very easy for the doctor and very difficult for the woman." It's easy for the doctor because it's quick and simple, the bread-and-butter surgery for many an OB/GYN. For the woman it's a major surgery in which an important organ is removed. Side effects can include adhesions and scars that cause chronic pain; lower back pain for months or years; lack of sexual sensation; bladder prolapse and almost always, months of painful recovery and hormone deficiencies and imbalances.

Women who have had a hysterectomy may be offered conventional estrogen replacement therapy to help relieve symptoms of surgical menopause, but it makes no sense to only replace estrogen. Both estrogen and progesterone, and often testosterone, are needed for hormone balance.

The ovaries and fallopian tubes

The ovaries sit about an inch away from the uterus on either side. They are very important organs of libido before menopause because they manufacture the hormones that orchestrate reproduction: estrogen, progesterone and testosterone. After menopause, they shrink, going from the size of walnuts to the size of almonds. At menopause, progesterone levels drop by 60 percent or more, estrogen by 40 percent, and testosterone by 30 percent. By the mid-60s, the ovaries are primarily producing androgens, or male hormones, and may continue this well into the 70s. You'll learn more about the production and roles of ovarian hormones in Chapter 4.

Polycystic ovary syndrome (PCOS) can dampen libido simply due to chronic ovarian pain. I'll go into the causes of PCOS and how to resolve it in Chapter 5.

The Orchestration of Libido

Brain, senses, skin, vulva, clitoris, vagina, G-spot, cervix, uterus and ovaries: all of these organs help to orchestrate libido. Restoring libido may involve focusing on one or more of them—making sure each is in a state of balanced health, exploring them more deeply or in new ways, talking with your partner about how you wish to explore them, and seeking out new ways to find and enhance sexual drive and pleasure. Future chapters will fill in important blanks about the role of hormone balance, bioidentical hormone therapy, awareness practices, and diet and supplements in nourishing these organs of desire and promoting their best possible function.

PART II

The Libido
Restoration Kit

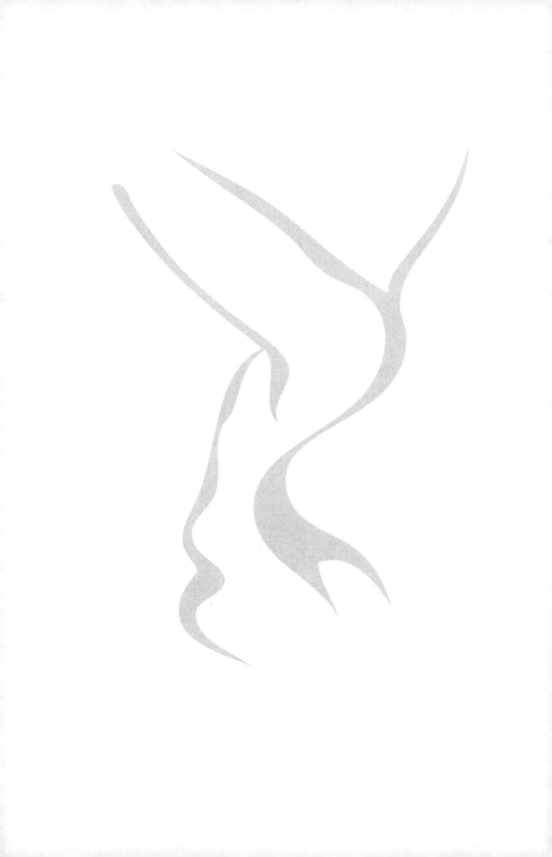

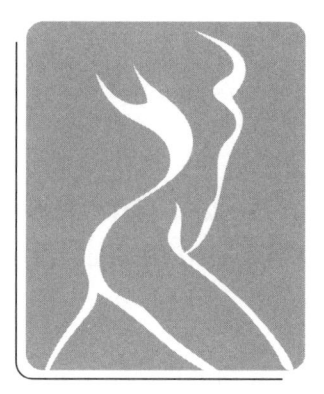

CHAPTER 4

Sexuality and Hormones – An Overview

I t's tough being a woman. With all of our cycles, secretions and hormonal fluctuations, we're always dealing with some female discomfort or other. And all this makes us an awful bother to our men.

At least, this is how it would seem to anyone whose only exposure to modern womanhood came through advertisements from the 1960s, 1970s and 1980s. A few choice quotes:

"It's not easy being a woman. Especially when you're a teenager." (From an ad for tampons.)

"Beware the one intimate neglect that can engulf you in marital grief." (For Lysol, in the days when it was used as a douche.)

"Almost any tranquilizer will calm her down…but at this age, estrogen may be what she really needs." (For Premarin, the first estrogen replacement drug.)

"He's suffering from estrogen deficiency. She is the reason why." (Again, for Premarin.)

Any woman who looks at those ads today will probably shake her head in disbelief, relieved at how far we've come since then, yet we're still being sold the idea that being a woman is difficult.

Yes: menstruation, pregnancy, childbirth, nursing, mothering, premenopause, perimenopause and menopause are experiences specific to the females of our species, any of which can bring challenges for us and the people we care about. All of the physical challenges associated with being female have hormone imbalances as the bottom line cause, but there are myriad factors, from stress and diet, to pesticides and insomnia that can affect hormone balance. Many doctors want to "fix" female hormone imbalances with a pill or a surgery—a birth control pill, an antidepressant, a hysterectomy, a cone biopsy—but in truth, most of us can restore balance with some basic lifestyle changes.

Around the time we begin to move into the 'tween' years at age 10 or so, hormones begin to change the way our bodies feel and work. Most of us can plan to ride those hormonal ebbs and flows for another 40 or so years, until well after menopause. After menopause our hormone levels are lower and steadier, but many of us miss the benefits of hormones. As our bodies age, glands age, and they can become less efficient at maintaining hormone balance.

Previous chapters have explored some of the physical and psychological influences that can cause libido to drop or disappear. In this chapter, you'll learn about the role female hormones can play in this dynamic.

Hormones: An Introduction

A hormone is a chemical messenger made in one of the many endocrine glands of the body—the ovaries, testicles, adrenals, thyroid, parathyroid and pancreas. Hormones are microscopic molecules, but they are incredibly potent. They have effects in concentrations of millionths of a gram. Shifts and changing relationships between hormones—both in monthly cycles and over ages and stages of the female life span can affect health, mood, libido, sexual response and overall well-being.

Our focus here will be estrogen, progesterone and testosterone, the so-called sex hormones made in the ovaries and adrenals. I'll also explain how thyroid hormones and cortisol interact with these hormones.

Ovaries, testicles, adrenals and thyroid glands receive signals from a gland found in the brain called the *pituitary,* which is also known as the "master gland" because of its role in regulating levels of most of the hormones in the body. When stimulated by a part of the brain called the *hypothalamus,* the pituitary makes a handful of signaling hormones that go out into the bloodstream. These hormones then trigger the endocrine glands to make *their* hormones, which also go out into the bloodstream to travel around in the body.

Estrogen, progesterone and testosterone then lock onto *receptor sites* on cells, which triggers cellular changes. The reproductive organs and the organs of libido contain lots of receptor sites for estrogens, progesterone and/ or testosterone, and so when those hormones are circulating, they preferentially affect those tissues.

Estrogens: Feminizing, Growth-Promoting

Estrogens are hormones made in the bodies of humans and animals, but this term also encompasses human-made estrogens (such as those found in birth control pills and hormone replacement), plant estrogens (e.g. those found in soybeans and red clover) and xenoestrogens (found in plastics, household chemicals, pesticides, etc.).

Estrogens made by the human body—also known as *endogenous* estrogens—promote cell growth. At puberty, they stimulate the creation of female breasts and hips, increase body fat and start the menstrual cycle. Estrogens are the drivers of the buildup of blood in the uterine lining that is either shed during menstruation or built up into a placenta during pregnancy. They also cause women to have higher vocal pitch and softer skin compared to men. Although estrogens aren't a direct driver of libido, lack of estrogen can cause vaginal dryness and atrophy, which can make sexual intercourse painful. When in the right balance, estrogens benefit bone health, mood, memory, sexual function, skin and energy levels.

Most of our estrogens are made in the ovaries, but also in the placenta (during pregnancy), breasts and adrenal glands. Women also make male hormones, and fat cells will transform them into estrogens. This is particularly true of belly fat, which is the primary provider of estrogen in a menopausal woman.

A woman who is underweight or doing strenuous exercise (e.g. a marathon runner) may make so little estrogen that she stops having periods. She may be unable to get pregnant or might show other signs of estrogen lack such as vaginal dryness or the beginnings of osteoporosis. A woman who is overweight, on the other hand may make too much estrogen, creating an imbalance with its complementary hormone, progesterone. Weight gain during the menopausal transition may actually be the body's way of making enough estrogen to maintain bone strength and mental sharpness!

A woman's body makes three main kinds of estrogen: *estradiol, estriol* and *estrone.* Estradiol is the primary estrogen in a premenopausal, non-pregnant woman. Estriol predominates during pregnancy and is important for vaginal health. Estrone is primarily an intermediate hormone, made from other hormones such as DHEA or testosterone, and then almost immediately converted to estradiol.

Each type of estrogen varies in terms of how *estrogenic* it is—meaning that some are more growth-promoting and generally more potent than others. In excess, estrogens can stimulate cancer growth. Estriol is the weakest and least estrogenic of the three endogenous estrogens; estrone holds the middle ground; and estradiol is the most strongly estrogenic.

When measured in saliva, normal, optimal levels of estradiol in a premenopausal woman during the luteal phase of the menstrual cycle (when ovulation occurs) are between 1.3 and 3.3 picograms per milliliter (pg/ml). In menopausal women who choose to try hormone replacement, our goal with estrogen is to restore that premenopausal range.

All hormones, including estrogens, are eventually *metabolized* (broken down) by enzymes in the liver. The synthetic estrogens and progestins in hormonal birth control affect the way estrogens are processed in the body. Genetics, lifestyle choices, environmental exposures and diet also impact estrogen metabolism. For example, eating a healthier diet that includes plenty of fiber and cruciferous vegetables is one way to shift estrogen metabolism in the direction of cancer *prevention*—toward weaker forms of estrogen and inactive breakdown products that are harmless. This will also aid in creating pro-libido hormone balance.

Many of the chemicals used to make household cleansers, solvents, building materials, pesticides, herbicides, non-stick cookware, air fresheners, plastics and beauty products contain estrogen-mimicking chemicals that enter the body and alter hormone activity and balance from an early age—potentially beginning before birth. Although one can't live in a modernized society without some exposure to these kinds of chemicals, knowing how to avoid them as much as possible—and how to use gentle methods to regain balance in the face of inevitable environmental exposures—is part of the big picture of hormone health. *This is covered in more depth in Chapter 9.*

Estrogens and mood

Too much or too little estrogen can have an effect on moods in some women, which can certainly contribute to low libido. If a woman is frazzled, frustrated, fatigued, irritated or anxious, she's not going to want to be sexual!

Estrogens raise levels of the mood-boosting neurotransmitters serotonin, dopamine and beta-endorphins. They also enhance production of acetylcholine and norepinephrine, neurotransmitters that help with quick thinking, attention and good memory. The brain's ability to make new connections is also enhanced by estrogens. When estrogens aren't balanced by adequate progesterone, estrogens can be *over*stimulating, leading to irritability, anxiety and insomnia.

Progesterone: Menstrual Timing, Estrogen Balancing, Pregnancy Maintenance

Progesterone plays a role in the timing of the menstrual cycle and helps to balance out the growth-promoting effects of estrogens. Like estrogen, it has effects throughout the body, on bone, blood vessels, mood, tissue growth and repair, fluid balance and nerve transmission. Progesterone and estrogen have many complementary effects.

For example:

- Part of estrogen's job during the first half of the menstrual cycle is to 'wake up' progesterone receptors so that progesterone can have optimal effect when it's produced after ovulation.

- Progesterone blunts the growth-promoting effect of estrogens.

- Estrogen is stimulating to the nervous system; progesterone is calming.

- Progesterone helps prevent excess tissue buildup in the uterus during the estrogen-stimulated proliferative (building-up) phase of the menstrual cycle.

- Progesterone helps protect the breasts against estrogen-stimulated tissue overgrowth that can lead to breast fibrocystic breasts or breast cancer.

This hormone also promotes better thyroid function and aids in balancing blood sugars, preventing water retention, building bone and reducing anxiety.

Ovulation occurs when an ovary releases an egg into the fallopian tube. Once the egg is on its way to the uterus, progesterone is produced. Progesterone levels rise and then fall through the 12 days following ovulation. During this *luteal phase* of the menstrual cycle, sex drive and pleasure in sex tend to rise, partly due to this rise in progesterone. A premenopausal woman's progesterone levels are normal if they're between 75 and 270 pg/ml (in saliva). As women age, less progesterone is produced, causing *luteal insufficiency*, which can cause estrogen dominance and infertility. Estrogen dominance also contributes to premenstrual syndrome (PMS). In younger women, luteal insufficiency can be caused by stress, poor diet and over-exercising.

If the egg is fertilized, progesterone production continues; if it isn't, estrogen and progesterone production drop and the uterine lining is shed in a menstrual period. After the first trimester of pregnancy, the placenta takes over progesterone production. By the end of pregnancy, the placenta is making 300 to 350 milligrams (mg) of progesterone a day—way up from the usual 15-20 mg produced per day in a normal menstrual cycle. Some of my patients say this phase of pregnancy is the best they have ever felt. Once the baby is born, progesterone and estrogen levels drop. Women who breastfeed will have lowered hormone levels for weeks to months. *See Chapter 11 for more on this.*

Estrogen Dominance: An Introduction

As women move into their late 30s and 40s, overall progesterone levels may fall while estrogens are still high—in part, due to more frequent *anovulatory cycles*, where ovulation and its accompanying surge of progesterone do not occur or there is luteal insufficiency (lower than optimal progesterone production). Enough estrogen is produced to build up the uterine lining and menstruation still takes place, but for that cycle, the ratio of estrogen to progesterone is skewed. Estrogen levels aren't necessarily too high, and may even be below the optimum, but without the natural balancing effect of progesterone, estrogen's impact is greater. During menopause, when ovulation stops completely, estrogens may remain high enough to perpetuate this imbalance. This imbalance in the estrogen-to-progesterone ratio is called *estrogen dominance*, a term coined by Dr. John Lee, author of *What Your Doctor May Not Tell You about Menopause*, a book I recommend that every woman over 40 have on her bookshelf!

Here is Dr. Lee's list of symptoms and conditions associated with estrogen dominance.

Symptoms and Conditions Associated With Estrogen Dominance

Acceleration of the aging process

Allergies, including asthma, hives, rashes, sinus congestion

Autoimmune disorders such as lupus erythematosis
and thyroiditis, and possibly Sjoegren's disease

Breast cancer

Breast tenderness

Cervical dysplasia (may cause a positive Pap smear)

Cold hands and feet (a symptom of thyroid dysfunction)

Copper excess

Decreased sex drive

Depression with anxiety or agitation

Dry eyes

Early onset of menopause

Endometrial (uterine) cancer

Fat gain, especially around the abdomen, hips and thighs

Fatigue

Fibrocystic breasts

Foggy thinking

Gallbladder disease

Hair Loss

Headaches

Hypoglycemia

Increased blood clotting (increasing risk of strokes)

Infertility

Irregular menstrual periods

Irritability

Insomnia

Magnesium deficiency

Memory loss

Mood swings

Osteoporosis

Polycystic ovaries

Premenopausal bone loss

PMS

Sluggish metabolism

Thyroid dysfunction mimicking hypothyroidism

Uterine fibroids

Water retention, bloating

Zinc deficiency

(From John Lee MD and Virginia Hopkins' *What Your Doctor May not Tell You About Menopause* [Warner Books 2004] reprinted with permission.)

Anovulatory cycles aren't the only factor in creating estrogen dominance. Other influences include:

- Being overweight or obese, which increases estrogen production

- Shifts in cortisol, insulin and adrenaline caused by chronic stress, which will also shift hormone balance in the direction of estrogen dominance

- Xenoestrogens from solvents, cleaning products, cosmetics, body care products, weed killers, sunscreens, insecticides, paints, dyes and building materials

Some xenoestrogens have weak estrogenic effects, while some exert much stronger effects—strong enough to contribute to estrogen dominance, and sometimes even strong enough to be carcinogenic. We're all exposed to these chemicals, which add to our overall estrogen burden. Recent research shows that xenoestrogens are present in the bodies of newborn babies. Even men can become estrogen dominant from living in this environmental soup of synthetic estrogens. In women, infertility and low progesterone production may be a result of these lifelong exposures. In men, it can result in obesity, low sperm count and prostate enlargement.

Chronic stress and adrenal fatigue—discussed in depth in Chapter 8—are major causes of low progesterone levels in women in their 40s. Cortisol, the hormone produced by the adrenals in response to stress, and progester-one are both built from the same precursor: a hormone called pregneno-lone. During chronic stress, the adrenals produce excess cortisol until they get tired and cortisol production drops. When this happens, the body tries to keep up with demand by shunting more pregnenolone into cortisol pro-duction, which means less raw material for the building of progesterone. This is known as "progesterone steal."

This makes perfect biological sense: if a woman's stress response system doesn't work properly, her body is in no condition to carry, bear or care for a child. She becomes functionally infertile until her body has regained bal-ance. Low progesterone levels make conception much less likely. For most women, returning to balance requires stress management and reduction.

Estrogen dominance, libido and the pill

One of the first things the average physician will do to treat a woman who shows up with PMS or difficult, irregular, painful or heavy periods—classic symptoms of estrogen dominance—is to prescribe birth control pills in an effort to "regulate her cycles." The same often happens to women in the years just before menopause.

Birth control pills (oral contraceptives) contain potent synthetic hormones that shut down the body's natural production of estrogens and proges-terone. The synthetic hormones may initially soothe symptoms, but over time are likely to make estrogen dominance symptoms worse. Birth control pills further decrease libido by raising levels of a biochemical called sex hormone-binding globulin (SHBG), which binds to hormones and makes them unavailable. This, in effect, lowers hormone levels, and testosterone in particular.

Women who don't require birth control may be given the estrogen Prema-rin and a progestin, the combination historically prescribed by doctors to women during and after menopause. The dosages are lower than those of birth control pills, but this combination of synthetic hormones can also suppress sex drive.

In contrast, bioidentical hormones applied transdermally (through the skin in gels, creams or patches) do not raise SHBG levels.

Testosterone: The Hormone of Libido

Men make about ten times more testosterone than women. Some women make considerably more testosterone than others. Normal testosterone levels for a premenopausal woman range between 16 to 55 pg/ml in saliva—a broad range.

A woman who is muscular and hard-driving is likely to have higher testosterone than a woman who's curvy and maternal. A woman with *too much* testosterone will develop acne and gain weight. She may lose her hair, or may grow hair where she doesn't want it. Some young women develop a syndrome called PCOS (polycystic ovary syndrome), where high insulin levels trigger excess testosterone production in the ovaries, which leads to the formation of ovarian cysts. Shifting to a diet that reduces insulin levels and helps shed excess body fat will help to re-balance hormones in women with PCOS.

During a woman's reproductive life and through menopause, testosterone is produced by the ovaries and adrenal glands. Levels fall gradually from a woman's 20s on. Testosterone has the strongest effect on libido of all of the hormones described here, which is why I've devoted a chapter to it. It has been called "the hormone of desire" because it's the primary driver of libido in both men and women. The next chapter covers testosterone in much more detail.

Thyroid Hormones and Adrenal Function

Thyroid hormones and the adrenal hormone cortisol aren't sex hormones, but they can shift and fall out of balance in response to the stress and as part of the aging process. Out-of-balance thyroid hormones and cortisol can directly affect libido, or can indirectly affect it by impacting sex hormone production and activity.

Thyroid hormones control metabolic rate—the rate at which the body's cells break down food and 'burn' it as fuel. It's estimated that one in ten Americans is affected by a thyroid hormone imbalance. Most are affected by an *underactive* thyroid gland that doesn't make enough of its hormones to sustain energy. Cold hands and feet, feelings of being cold, dry skin and hair, joint aches and pains, muscle cramps, weak muscles and weight gain of five or more pounds without change in diet can be due to low thyroid hormone. Much rarer is *overactive* thyroid, a condition called Graves' disease that has to be treated medically. It causes the opposite symptom profile: mania, fast heartbeat, a feeling of being overheated and weight loss. Low thyroid can cause low libido; Graves' disease can make libido excessive.

Thyroid deficiency can contribute to heavy periods, brain fog and overall lack of energy—all symptoms associated with estrogen dominance. Estrogen dominance can't be completely resolved if thyroid issues are still present, and likewise, thyroid issues in women cannot be completely resolved without addressing estrogen dominance.

Standard testing of thyroid hormone levels often only measures thyroid stimulating hormone (TSH), which rises when thyroid function falls in an effort to get the thyroid to make more hormone. The range for "normal" TSH in a blood test is huge, between 0.4 and 4.5 milli-international units per liter. A woman can have normal TSH but still be hypothyroid, or thyroid deficient.

I give thyroid hormone even to people with mild deficiencies to bring them up to an optimal range. This is something that can only be done with a doctor's help; thyroid hormone is available only by prescription.

Cortisol and Adrenal Fatigue

Cortisol is a hormone produced by the adrenal glands. It's produced in response to stress, and it helps the body to adapt by raising blood pressure and altering circulation to bring more blood flow and oxygen to muscles, increasing breathing and heart rate, and sharpening attention. When life is stressful for years or decades, the adrenals can get tapped out. They lose their ability to keep up with life's demands. The result is what's known as *adrenal fatigue.*

Symptoms of adrenal fatigue can be confused with symptoms of hypothyroidism or other hormone imbalances:

- Allergies to things you were never allergic to before
- Anxiety, depression
- Chemical sensitivity (e.g. reactions to perfumes, cleaning products, etc.)
- Craving for sweets and salt
- Difficulty falling asleep
- Fatigue in the middle of the day
- Feeling cold
- More frequent infections
- Waking up in the middle of the night

If a woman has been living in a stressed-out state, her adrenals may get tired and unable to make enough cortisol to keep up with demand. (Adrenal exhaustion that may be life-threatening is called Addison's disease.) Testing of adrenal hormone levels can help determine whether adrenal fatigue is dampening libido. In Chapter 8 you'll learn about ways to counter adrenal fatigue, as well as ways to calm adrenal function in the context of a stressful life (and whose life isn't stressful nowadays?).

Hormones Through a Woman's Ages and Stages

Even in the womb, we're strongly impacted by hormones. All fetuses start out female. In a fetus with a Y chromosome, testosterone kicks in to turn what would otherwise become a clitoris, labia, ovaries and uterus into a penis, testicles and prostate gland. Without that Y chromosome, estrogen is the predominant hormone affecting a female fetus' development. Her reproductive organs form, complete with hundreds of thousands of tiny ova (eggs) in the ovaries, very early in her fetal life. At birth, it's not unusual for both female and male babies to have swollen breasts and even a tiny bit of milk in their breasts. This is the effect of hormones from the mother's body.

Let's look at how hormones continue to ebb, flow and interact through the female lifespan as she moves through childhood, adolescence, young adulthood and middle age, and on into her later years. In Part III we'll go into greater detail about ages and stages from the 20s forward—how libido can be maintained or increased and how to achieve healthy balance in the face of the unique challenges of each stage of life.

Infancy, childhood and puberty

Levels of estrogen, testosterone and progesterone are very low from birth until puberty. In the two to three years before puberty, the adrenals begin to make more DHEA—a shift known as *adrenarche*. This triggers the budding of breasts in girls. Pubic hair, underarm hair and thicker leg hair may begin to appear around this time. Then, at puberty, estrogen levels begin to rise, leading into the first period (menarche).

Ovulation might occur with the first period, or it can be delayed for months or years after periods begin—which means that little to no progesterone is made to balance out the estrogens that create the menstrual cycle. The next time you find yourself shaking your head over the incredible mood swings of a young teen girl, remember that she might be dealing with the same hormone imbalances that can arise in the years before menopause!

The 20s and early 30s

In a woman's 20s and early 30s, her hormonal rhythms hit their stride. These are her years of peak fertility, and for most, libido is strongest in this decade. Hormone imbalances may be a factor when lack of libido, PMS, endometriosis, painful periods, painful or lumpy breasts, very heavy menstrual flow, uterine fibroids, infertility, repeat miscarriages or symptoms of polycystic ovary syndrome (PCOS) are present. These imbalances are usually about estrogen dominance due to low progesterone production. High levels of stress can create or worsen this imbalance. Hormone testing and balancing with a physician who's skilled in these areas can help tremendously with these health issues.

Premenopause: Mid-30s through mid-40s

The hormonal shifts that occur between a woman's mid-30s to her late 40s are a precursor to those that occur right around the time of menopause. Dr. John Lee distinguished this stage of life from *perimenopause* by giving it a different name: *premenopause*. Perimenopause describes the year or two just before menopause, when estrogen, progesterone and testosterone all drop as periods come less frequently and then stop. Premenopause describes hormonal shifts that can begin in the mid-30s, as much as 20 years before menopause itself.

As early as the mid-30s, many women begin to have more *anovulatory* (no ovulation) menstrual cycles, and the consequence is that little or no progesterone is produced. Even ovulatory cycles may produce less progesterone than they once did.

Estrogen dominance in a premenopausal woman may show up as worsening PMS, difficult or irregular periods, mood swings, mental fogginess, fat gain in the abdomen and hips, headaches, bloating, fluid retention, a chronically red face, anxiety, depression, fatigue, sudden worsening of allergies, asthma, skin problems and sinus congestion.

I see many women who are in this stage of life. A pattern has emerged among these patients, and I can see it clearly within minutes of sitting down to talk in our initial appointment. I call them "frazzled women."

The Frazzled Woman

Many women in their 30s and 40s end up feeling completely stressed out by the combination of life challenges and physical symptoms that come with estrogen dominance. They get to the point of operating from this place of frazzled-ness—where they are very stressed even when life isn't particularly stressful. When there *is* real stress, they feel completely overwhelmed. Women who fall into this category tend to be curvier and hippier—their bodies show that they have higher levels of estrogen than women who are thin and muscular (who are likely to have lower estrogen and higher testosterone). These curvier women tend to have more problem with estrogen dominance in premenopause, and they also tend to have more severe menopausal symptoms as estrogen levels drop.

The frazzled woman has gained weight and her skin doesn't look healthy. She can't concentrate—in fact, she can't even read a book anymore. She's irritable. The kids annoy her. If she's still in a marriage, she's having relationship problems because she's irritable toward her husband. Her energy is low and her libido is sapped. She just does what she has to in order to get through the day, get through work and get through taking care of the kids. When she finally gets to bed she passes out, exhausted, but then can't sleep through the night.

Over time, she loses the drive to put time or energy into preparing healthy, nutritious meals for herself and her family. Her irritability precludes her asking her partner or kids for more help with cooking and home care. She'll start to rely on fast food and prepared foods, which are likely to put extra pounds on her and make her feel even less healthy. As she grumpily buckles down and tries to keep doing it all herself, she gets more and more resentful. She stops exercising because she doesn't have the energy anymore. Is it any surprise that a woman in this state doesn't have much interest in sex?

With most frazzled women the first things we address are slow but sure step-by-step changes to a healthier lifestyle. I nearly always prescribe bioidentical progesterone (more on this in a bit). After a few months I see their families at soccer practice or ballet class and they tell me, "Thank you so much for giving us our Mom back." The de-frazzled woman is more balanced and less irritable. She can read a book, sit down, focus and concentrate without feeling constantly scattered. It's not that she has any less to do in life, she just doesn't feel as stressed about it. Her short-term memory is back, her energy starts to return, and she sleeps through the night. And last but not least, her libido begins to reappear. This makes her husband happier, which makes her and the kids happier.

Perimenopause and menopause

In the mid-to-late 40s, the classic symptoms of oncoming menopause arrive: hot flashes, night sweats, insomnia, vaginal dryness, weight gain, mood swings, and skin changes. Periods get erratic and then, finally, they stop altogether. The Change is in progress. For about 40 percent of women these changes are severe enough to seek medical help.

By menopause, which is defined as one year after your last period, estrogen levels have fallen 60 to 80 percent and progesterone is almost nonexistent;

it is only being made in small amounts by the adrenal glands. However, the ovaries are still making male hormones (including testosterone), which are converted to estrogen by fat cells. Some women continue to make adequate testosterone through menopause; others notice a more distinct drop.

Low estrogen levels in perimenopause and post-menopause can lead to brain fog, hot flashes, depression, headaches, sleeplessness, memory lapses, urinary incontinence and lack of libido. The vagina begins to change, becoming drier, thinner and less sensitive.

Even if estrogen levels are adequate, low progesterone and testosterone levels can perpetuate imbalances that affect libido and well-being.

So, let's say you think you might be one of those frazzled women—and that a hormone imbalance may be contributing to your lack of libido. Or perhaps you're on the cusp of menopause or already in menopause, and you're experiencing classic menopausal symptoms, including lack of libido. What's next? It might be time to consider hormone testing and using bioidentical hormones to try to create hormone balance.

Bioidentical vs. Synthetic Hormones

Bioidentical hormones are carbon copies of the hormones made in your body. Synthetic hormones like the progestins used in most hormonal birth control and conventional hormone replacement therapy (HRT) have similarities to natural hormones, but they've had a few molecules tweaked and moved around in a laboratory in order to make the hormone into a drug that can be patented and sold for a high price in the competitive pharmaceutical market. Progestins are more potent than progesterone, and have many undesirable effects that progesterone does not.

The synthetic estrogens used in birth control pills and HRT are similarly the-same-but-different; they have some estrogen effects but not all, and an array of undesirable side effects. The most commonly prescribed estrogen for menopausal women for many years was Premarin.

What You Should Know About Using Bioidentical Hormones

Let's say your neighbor is on hormones and doing great; should you ask for the same protocol for yourself? Not at all! Every woman who comes into my office is unique, and the advice I give is different for everyone. Physicians have standard protocols and starting doses, but many factors need to be taken into account. For example if a woman has tired adrenals, I may not give her testosterone right off the bat. Each woman needs to be addressed differently according to past reactions to medications, baseline hormone levels and adrenal health. We can't prescribe bioidentical hormone replacement in a book. An individualized approach, with the help of a physician experienced with bioidenticals, is the ideal scenario. Although bioidentical progesterone creams are available over-the-counter (OTC), estrogens and testosterone are only available by prescription.

A premenopausal woman is not likely to need estrogens, but almost every woman with a hormone imbalance—pre-, peri-, or postmenopausal—benefits from progesterone. Some may need testosterone as well, which I can determine through hormone testing. Before menopause, progesterone helps maintain balance with estrogens and reduces symptoms of estrogen dominance; during and after the menopausal transition, when estrogens drop, it can optimize the effects of estrogen. Any time a woman uses estrogen replacement therapy, progesterone needs to be given to maintain hormone balance. Let me phrase that differently because it's so important—*every* woman taking estrogen should also be using progesterone.

Progesterone in a *transdermal* form (given as a cream, absorbed through the skin) works well for many women. Women who have lots of stress and need help sleeping—who almost always turn out to have tired adrenals—often benefit more from oral progesterone. When oral progesterone is processed in the liver, it creates metabolites, or byproducts, that help with sleep. Just getting good sleep solves a lot of the issues that cause libido to drop.

Premenopausal women who use progesterone should do so only during the luteal phase. If symptoms are severe and estrogen dominance is pronounced, I sometimes use a half-strength dose from days five through 11 of the cycle, and then full-strength from days 12 to 28 of the cycle. (Day one of the menstrual cycle is the first day of menstrual bleeding.)

Women who have symptoms of estrogen deficiency can use transdermal estrogens (in patches or creams). I almost always use a combination of estradiol and estriol. If vaginal dryness and atrophy are the only symptoms of estrogen deficiency, I have women apply estrogen cream directly to the vagina.

How about DHEA?

One hormone that's widely available over the counter is *dehydroepiandrosterone*, or DHEA, which can be transformed into estrogens, testosterone and progesterone in the body. Should you consider supplementing with DHEA instead of going to the trouble of visiting a doctor for a more detailed prescription? I don't recommend this, and here's why.

There's no way to control how DHEA is transformed in the body. In one woman, it might help to create better hormone balance; in another, it might worsen imbalances. DHEA is best taken under physician supervision, where adjustments can be made if imbalances seem to get worse. I often prescribe it when adrenal fatigue is part of the picture, but because I monitor hormone levels, I can adjust the dose if DHEA begins to worsen symptoms of estrogen dominance or seems to raise testosterone levels high enough to cause symptoms like growth of facial hair or acne.

Summing Up: Hormones, Libido, and Quality of Life

Many women show up at my office believing that all they'll need to do to solve their libido problem is balance their hormones. Although this is sometimes true, it more often is not.

Restoring libido almost always involves more than hormone balancing. It's a good place to start, though. You might compare balanced hormones with an artist's canvas: without a clean, well-stretched and prepared canvas, the artist will find it much more challenging to create her best work. And without the backdrop of hormone balance, a woman will find it more difficult to restore her libido. Understanding and achieving hormone balance will make the other steps described in this book easier to take.

Changing diet, lifestyle and stress coping skills can also shift hormone balance. Even if you'd rather not use bioidentical hormones, good hormone balance and libido can be restored through other means. The foods we eat, the thoughts we think, the way we relate with our partners, how we cope with stress, whether we get enough exercise and sleep—all of these factors are just as important as bioidentical hormones, if not more so, to restoring libido.

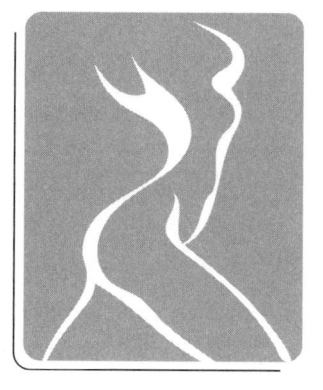

CHAPTER 5

Testosterone – The Hormone of Arousal

A s Ellie and Dan entered their 60s and looked forward to retirement, Ellie often found herself feeling irritated with Dan's continuing desire to have sex. "I thought I was done with all that," she said. "Why can't he slow down too? I'm perfectly OK with not having sex, but he's not." Ellie finally came to see me about resurrecting her libido, not for herself, but for her husband. She was skeptical but willing to give bioidentical hormones, including testosterone, a try. Three months later Ellie returned for a follow-up visit with a sheepish grin and admitted, "I can't believe it, you've given me back my sex life. My husband is so happy and so am I!" She explained that a year ago they had gone on a cruise to the Caribbean and it had been an unhappy trip because she wasn't interested in sex and felt unfairly pressured by Dan. They had recently gone on another cruise, to Europe, and this time she said, "It was just fabulous. I'm having sex with my husband again and I want it as much as he does. But the best part is that we're laughing and having fun together again because the sex brought us closer, back to a more intimate relationship."

We could have named this chapter Testosterone — Not Just for Men! Although testosterone levels are highest in men, it's an equally important hormone in women, and an essential part of a healthy libido for both sexes. That being said, it's important to keep in mind throughout this chapter that testosterone is the hormone of *physical* arousal. If the mental and emotional *desire* to have sex isn't there, all the testosterone in the world isn't going to restore a lost libido. And if emotional issues in a relationship cause a lack of libido, testosterone may restore only the lost libido, which may then be directed at someone outside the relationship.

The women I see who most need testosterone are those who have had a hysterectomy and had their ovaries removed. That's a very abrupt, drastic change because hormone levels pretty much fall off a cliff. A woman in her 30s or 40s whose libido has been fine will come to see me after having her uterus and ovaries removed and say "Oh my God, I opened my eyes after the surgery and things were never the same again." Most of those women do very well just by replacing what they've lost with bioidentical hormones, usually estrogen, progesterone and testosterone.

The Biochemistry of Testosterone

Testosterone is an *androgen*, or male hormone, but women also make it in small amounts, just as men make estrogen in small amounts. In a woman, testosterone is manufactured in the adrenal glands, the ovaries and the fat cells, and it peaks in her 20s. Then, like the other hormones, testosterone levels decline with age, but not as much as estrogen and progesterone. In fact, a woman's ovaries and adrenal glands may continue to manufacture testosterone through her 70s and beyond. The Rancho Bernardo Study showed that bioavailable or free testosterone levels in women *increased* with age, "…reaching premenopausal levels for the 70–79 decade with relatively stable levels thereafter."

In women, approximately 25 percent of testosterone is made by the ovaries, 25 percent is made by the adrenal glands, and 50 percent is made by conversion of androstenedione (an androgen) or DHEA in body fat. Androstenedione is derived equally from adrenals and the ovaries, which means that overall, about half of a woman's testosterone comes from her ovaries. The total daily testosterone production in premenopausal women is about 300 to 500 micrograms (0.3 to 0.5 mg). When circulating in blood, about 80 percent of the testosterone is bound to sex hormone binding globulin (SHBG), and another 19 percent is bound to albumin, leaving only 1 percent that is unbound or "free." Only the free testosterone can be used by the body.

In some women, testosterone may quickly be converted to the estrogen known as estradiol, which can cause estrogen dominance symptoms such as breast tenderness and weight gain. *Chapter 6 has suggestions for blocking this conversion.*

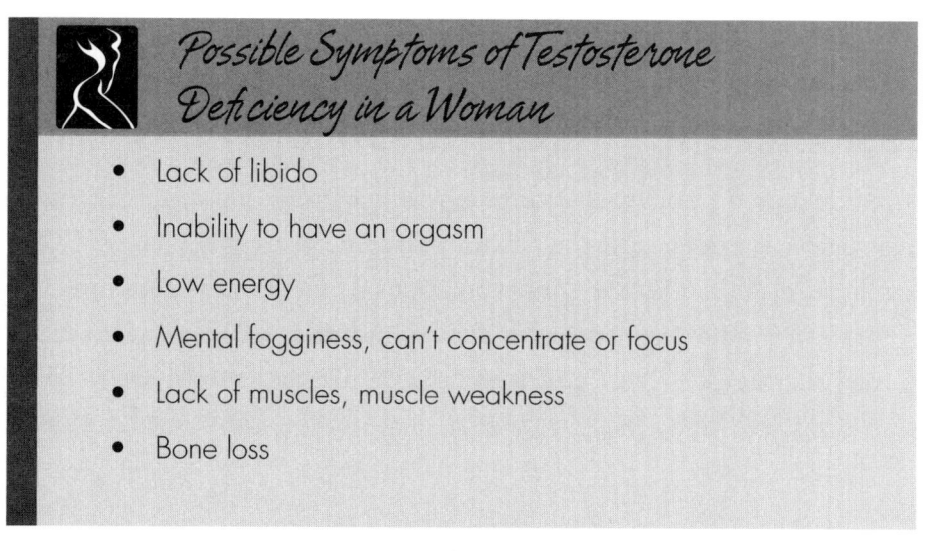

Possible Symptoms of Testosterone Deficiency in a Woman

- Lack of libido
- Inability to have an orgasm
- Low energy
- Mental fogginess, can't concentrate or focus
- Lack of muscles, muscle weakness
- Bone loss

- Slow metabolism, easily gains weight
- Cries easily, "at the least little thing"
- Easily offended, oversensitive
- Depression
- Fearfulness, timidity, afraid to try new things
- Prolapsed organs—uterus, bladder
- Urinary incontinence

Women with an *excess* of testosterone may have symptoms of hair loss on the head, excessive hair growth on the rest of the body, acne, polycystic ovary syndrome (PCOS), and irritability or "testiness." Testosterone is an "upper," in that it increases energy, but in doing so it will rev up the adrenals, which can be counter-productive in women who have tired adrenals. It's like revving your car in neutral. Using supplemental testosterone causes the adrenals to try to rev up, but if you don't have enough adrenal reserve you'll feel worse. If you have a little bit of adrenal reserve you'll feel great for a little while, but within four to six weeks you'll use up what you have, and then you'll crash.

Testosterone, PCOS and Heart Disease

Some doctors do not want to prescribe testosterone for women because they believe it can increase the risk for polycystic ovary syndrome (PCOS) and heart disease. There is confusion about women and testosterone because women who have polycystic PCOS and diabetes have higher-than-normal testosterone levels, and women with diabetes almost always have heart disease.

What the research shows is that women with a lot of fat around the middle, and existing diabetes and/or heart disease tend to have elevated testosterone levels. However, the high testosterone levels are caused by the obesity and diabetes, not the other way around. Testosterone is an anabolic hormone, which means that it builds muscle and bone, promotes good circulation and balances the effects of catabolic hormones such as insulin and cortisol. When we're eating too much sugar and refined carbohydrates and making too much insulin in response, the body tries to balance this out by making more testosterone. The same is true of cortisol; when we're stressed and our cortisol levels are chronically high, the body responds by producing more testosterone.

Research on women and testosterone has been further complicated by the use of synthetic testosterones such as methyltestosterone, and by the use of very high doses, both of which can be harmful. Like all hormones, both too little and too much testosterone can be harmful. As always, we're looking for balance.

Research done with women of normal weight who do not have diabetes or heart disease, and who are deficient in testosterone, shows that they benefit in many ways, including reduced heart disease risk factors, increased muscle mass and weight loss.

Women who miss testosterone

When hormones begin to decline with age, some women miss their testosterone a lot more than others. These women are what I call *testosterone dominant*. A testosterone dominant woman tends to have a slim, athletic build and tends to approach the world from a more logical and business-like point of view. For example, Susan is one of my testosterone-dominant patients who's a successful lawyer and executive and who travels for business. She's very lean, has small breasts and has a very confident, assertive personality. When she came to me for hormone balancing, she did not feel like herself until she was taking a relatively high dose of testosterone.

Testosterone also provides what's been called an emotional shield. Men don't cry nearly as much as women do, and it has a lot to do with testosterone. Perimenopausal women will say, "All of a sudden I cry at everything." This can be caused by hormonal fluctuations, by estrogen dominance, and by testosterone deficiency.

When we're suffering from long-term, chronic stress and tired adrenals, we outstrip our supply of cortisol, and so the body will sacrifice both progesterone and testosterone production in favor of cortisol. The way I view it is that when we outstrip our supply of cortisol, then the progesterone is sacrificed, and when we outstrip our supply of progesterone then our testosterone is sacrificed. I see so many perimenopausal women who are adrenally fatigued, estrogen dominant and testosterone deficient, all at the same time. These are the "frazzled" women that I described earlier.

When to Use Testosterone

Women who have had their ovaries removed benefit dramatically from testosterone replacement therapy, in their sense of well-being, improved muscle mass and a greatly improved sex life. This is well established by research; the famous Rancho Bernardo Study showed that women whose ovaries were removed had 40 percent lower testosterone levels than women of the same age who had their ovaries. But what about women who still have their ovaries yet have symptoms of low testosterone? The first step is to test hormone levels, and even then I don't rush to prescribe testosterone.

Even when testosterone levels test a bit low, when women are perimenopausal or menopausal, have gained some weight, feel tired all the time, haven't been eating well, and aren't exercising, I'll usually address lifestyle issues first before suggesting testosterone. These women are caught in that descending spiral in which hormone imbalance and stress cause fatigue, so they stop exercising and eat more junk food, so they gain weight and get even more tired, and meanwhile their self-esteem is also taking a dive.

Often, just adding progesterone to lifestyle changes is enough to restore libido. Progesterone supports the production of cortisol, balances the effects of estrogen, and has a calming effect that is helpful for women who are wired but tired. Most often, this approach restores testosterone levels.

Once we've got the lifestyle issues on the right track, giving testosterone to a woman who is truly deficient can really improve her metabolism, her energy, her libido and her outlook on life. Studies have shown that women who are treated with testosterone show an improvement in self-esteem.

How to use testosterone

Testosterone is available only by prescription. It comes in the form of injection, cream or gel, sublingual drops, oral tablets, pellets injected under the skin and troches (under the tongue). The creams and gels can be used on the skin or vaginally.

The ovaries of a premenopausal woman can make anywhere from 0.3 to 0.5 mg of testosterone daily, and therefore testosterone doses for women vary quite a lot, and vary by delivery method. For example, for a small woman who is not a testosterone dominant type of person and wants to use a cream or gel, I might start with 0.5 mg daily and work up or down from there as needed. Research has shown that a transdermal testosterone dose of just 0.15 mg of testosterone daily can increase levels of "free" testosterone five-fold. Because the amount of testosterone that a woman makes is so small, it doesn't take a large increase or decrease to have noticeable effects.

I'm very careful about how I use testosterone pellets because once the pellet is under the skin, it doesn't come out and it lasts for about three months. I've seen women with too much testosterone lose a lot of hair, get very anxious, have insomnia and become irritable. Excess testosterone can rev up the adrenal glands and ultimately cause fatigue, and it can be converted to estrogen and cause anxiety. When I notice these kinds of symptoms in women who are taking testosterone pellets, I'll give them some Chrysin, an herb that helps block the conversion of testosterone to estrogen. In women who aren't using pellets, when the symptoms arise the dose can be immediately lowered and symptoms rapidly resolve.

Testosterone injections can work very well for women who are willing to give themselves a sub-cutaneous injection once a week. The advantage of the injections is that a woman can easily and exactly raise or lower her dose depending on symptoms. For example, if she's growing a mustache and getting irritable she can lower the dose. If her energy and libido are flagging she can raise the dose.

When women are reluctant to take testosterone, I'll sometimes recommend that they try taking DHEA, a steroid hormone made primarily in the adrenal glands. In women who take DHEA supplements I find that it often raises testosterone levels, and sometimes raises estrogen levels. Women only need 5 to 10 mg daily of DHEA. Even at that low dose, it's a good idea to test hormone levels to make sure it's not raising estrogen levels too high. Women who take DHEA, which is available over-the-counter, should also always take progesterone with it, to balance any conversion to estrogen.

DHEA does not reliably and consistently raise testosterone and estrogen levels. The ideal approach to hormone balance is to supplement each hormone separately.

Testosterone—Approach with Caution

Testosterone can be a valuable piece in the libido restoration puzzle, but it needs to be treated with respect. It can be thrilling for a woman who has been feeling fearful, foggy, fatigued and sexless to suddenly (sometimes with four hours) feel confident, focused, energetic and sexy. But when overdone, testosterone can create anxiety, insomnia and irritability, and may cause estrogen dominance and increase risk factors for heart disease. Women using testosterone should test their hormone levels about every three months, and be aware of the symptoms of excess testosterone and estrogen dominance.

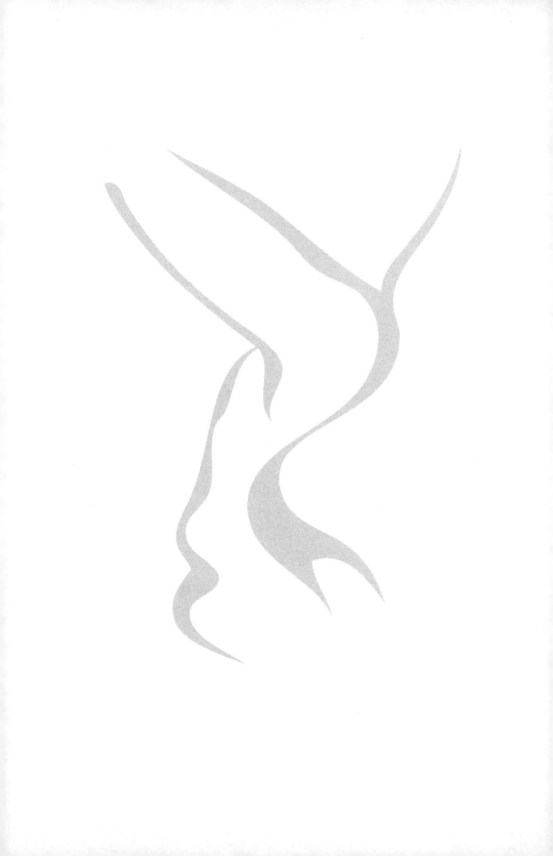

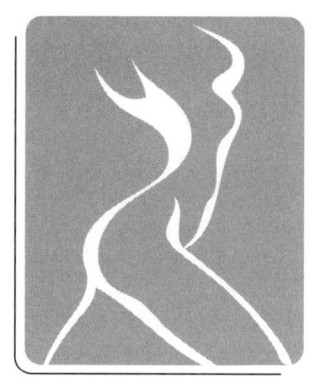

CHAPTER 6

My Favorite Libido-Boosting Supplements and Herbs

I sometimes recommend nutritional supplements and herbs for treatment of low libido. They're safe, gentle and effective for the woman who just needs a little boost to create some sexual heat.

Physically, sexual arousal takes place when the blood vessels of the genitals and other erogenous zones expand. As more blood flows into those areas, they swell and become more sensitive. Studies show that women watching erotic videos can become sexually aroused *without even knowing it*. The body is aroused but the brain is busy elsewhere. This is likely one of the reasons that research on herbal remedies for low libido has been mixed— it's difficult for researchers to measure desire.

Arousal originates in the erogenous zones; desire originates in the mind, emotions and imagination. Remember that in the quest to restore libido, we need to address both. If the herb or supplement doesn't help enhance your sex drive, it may be worth trying a different one, or it may be time to address your level of desire.

Herbs that increase libido are known as aphrodisiacs, and have been used for centuries, in every corner of the globe. The word aphrodisiac originates from Aphrodite, the Greek goddess of love and beauty.

Sexual Arousal is All about Blood Flow

Lack of arousal is clear cut in a man whose erections are soft or don't last. A fully aroused erection is all about good blood flow and, not surprisingly, a fully aroused woman is also all about good blood flow. Inadequate blood flow to a woman's genitals can't be easily seen, but she can feel it in the form of uncomfortable or even painful sex.

The herbs and supplements covered in this chapter enhance physical sexual arousal. *In Chapter 8 I'll share some secrets to enhancing awareness of arousal that in turn will enhance desire.*

Women with libido issues can try a variety of herbs and nutritional supplements that help make arousal occur more quickly and intensely by enhancing blood flow. Many of the herbs discussed in this chapter also affect hormones in ways that aid libido and arousal.

Be careful in your choice of herbs and herbal blends—look for a trusted brand. Some herbal aphrodisiac blends have been found to contain sildenafil, otherwise known as Viagra!

Begin With Good Cardiovascular Health

In general, blood circulation tends to become less efficient as we age. Cardiovascular disease, including peripheral vascular disease (where the small blood vessels that feed the extremities become clogged), is one of the most common health problems from midlife on. Men with erectile dysfunction often also have circulatory problems that set the stage for heart disease; the same can be true for women whose genital circulation is compromised.

To set a foundation for your body's best response to the supplements described in this chapter, take good care of your circulatory system by getting regular exercise, maintaining good eating habits and taking a multivitamin and fish oil as recommended in Chapter 9. Then, try adding one or a few supplements that can enhance arousal.

Recommended Supplements and Herbs for Arousal

While it's fine to take B vitamins along with any of the other herbal supplements, I recommend not trying more than two of the herbs at a time if you choose to use them separately. (Some of the products that show promise in research and in my practice contain combinations of libido-enhancing herbs and nutrients; this suggestion doesn't apply if you decide on one of these products.) That way, you can discern which herbs are most helpful in your own personal journey back to great sex. Unless otherwise stated, all of these herbs are fine for men to try, too.

Although nutrients like vitamins and minerals almost never interact adversely with prescription medications, herbs can and do interact with drugs. I'll address the most important of these interactions in this chapter, but if you take one or more prescription drugs every day, it's best to check with your pharmacist before starting a new herb to rule out any possibility of harmful interactions.

L-Arginine

Not only does the human circulatory system push blood through roughly 60,000 miles of blood vessels; not only does it manage to get needed oxygen and nutrients to every cell in the body—it can also change the relative amount of blood sent to different parts of the body according to need.

After a meal, for example, blood vessels that feed the muscular walls of the stomach and intestines expand to support good digestion. If, right after a meal, you realize you're late for an appointment a few blocks away and decide to jog over, blood supply to the digestive organs is reduced and vessels that feed the muscles open wide. Launching out of that post-lunch slump is possible because the body knows to send more oxygen-rich blood to wherever it's most needed. Arousal works the same way. As your body and brain together perceive that sex is on the horizon, blood flow is diverted to the genitals and other erogenous zones.

In response to changes in activity or environment, hormones and other body chemicals are produced and sent to circulate through the bloodstream. A substance called *nitric oxide* is formed in blood vessels in response. Nitric oxide has a *dilating* effect on blood vessels—it causes them to widen and allow more blood to flow through. Many drugs used to treat impotence and high blood pressure work by raising nitric oxide levels, and many herbs and foods that enhance arousal work through this same mechanism.

Nitric oxide is produced when a specific enzyme acts on an amino acid called L-arginine, which naturally exists throughout the human body. Research suggests that taking supplemental L-arginine will increase nitric oxide activity and thus enhance sexual arousal.

Arginine seems to work best when teamed up with other libido-enhancing supplements. A supplement called ArginMax, which contains L-arginine, ginseng, ginkgo, damiana and vitamins and minerals, has been studied at the University of Illinois and the University of Hawaii. In one study, 108 women—59 premenopausal, 20 perimenopausal and 29 postmenopausal—took ArginMax or a placebo for four weeks. Most of the premenopausal women using ArginMax reported substantial improvement in libido and sexual satisfaction after the four weeks were up. They desired sex more often and experienced greater overall satisfaction with their sex lives compared to the placebo group. The perimenopausal ArginMax group had more frequent sex and greater sexual satisfaction, plus some relief from vaginal dryness. In the postmenopausal group, 51 percent of those taking ArginMax reported increased sexual desire, while only 8 percent of the placebo group found themselves wanting more sex.

In another study, 77 women took either ArginMax or a placebo. Of those who took the supplement, 73.5 percent reported improvements in their sexual satisfaction (including better vaginal lubrication, more frequent intercourse and orgasm, and more intense clitoral sensation) compared with only 37.2 percent of the placebo group.

Arginine can also be applied directly to the clitoris to enhance sexual sensations and arousal. If your doctor is willing to prescribe it, you can have a compounding pharmacist make a preparation called Scream Cream, which contains non-prescription and prescription agents (L-arginine, aminophylline, isosorbid dinitrate, ergoloid mesylate and pentoxifylline). The drugs and nutrients are added to a cream base that promotes absorption of the amino acid into the body, where it dilates blood vessels.

Recommendations:

If arginine is taken alone, I recommend 2 to 3 grams (2,000 to 3,000 milligrams) of arginine per day. Take combination formulas like ArginMax according to package directions.

Precautions:

Do not take oral L-arginine if you have had a heart attack in the past few months. One study found an increased risk of death in patients who took arginine supplements in the months following a heart attack.

Do not take oral L-arginine if you have gastroesophageal reflux (GERD) or chronic heartburn. It can increase stomach acidity.

Do not use topical or oral L-arginine if you have genital or oral herpes or shingles. Arginine can increase the likelihood of flareups.

B vitamins

Some women feel too energy-depleted to follow through on even their best intentions to rev up their sex lives. When I see a patient who has just run out of gas, one of the first things I suspect is that she isn't getting enough B vitamins. Depression and bad PMS can also suggest a need for more vitamins in the B family.

B vitamins are needed to transform carbohydrates into energy at the cellular level. They are water-soluble, which means that the body can't store them; any extra you consume will be flushed out with urine. Regular intake is needed to keep levels of B vitamins high enough to ensure a steady supply of energy.

Birth control pills deplete the body of B vitamins. Women who use chemical contraceptives are at greater risk of B vitamin deficiency and are more likely to benefit from a supplement.

Recommendations

What I usually suggest is a multivitamin that contains approximately:

> 30 milligrams (mg) of vitamin B1 (thiamine)
>
> 35 mg of B2 (riboflavin)
>
> 80 mg of vitamin B3 (niacin)
>
> 80 mg of vitamin B5 (pantothenic acid)
>
> 40 mg of vitamin B6 (pyridoxine)
>
> 400 micrograms (mcg) of vitamin B9 (folic acid)

Higher doses of vitamin B6—300 milligrams daily for the week prior to menstruation—may be helpful for women with severe PMS.

Vitamin B12 is especially good for increasing energy, but it isn't well absorbed as an oral supplement. Try a sublingual (absorbed in tablet or lozenge form beneath the tongue) form that delivers 500 to 1000 micrograms (mcg) of vitamin B12 per day.

Precautions

The B vitamins are all safe to use even in doses far beyond what's recommended here. Any excess leaves the body through urine. No harmful interactions of B vitamins with drugs or herbs have been identified.

Damiana (turnera aphrodisiaca)

Indigenous people of Central and South America were the first to use the leaves of the plant damiana as an all-purpose medicine and as an aphrodisiac. Today, damiana is used worldwide as an herbal remedy for male infertility, menopause symptoms, headaches, constipation and bed-wetting, among other things.

Damiana is said to help enhance blood flow to the genital and urinary systems. Modern scientific research also reveals that damiana contains natural chemicals—including alkaloids, flavonoids, saponins and sterols—that gently influence hormone levels in both men and women to aid arousal and sex drive. Specifically, components of this herb block an enzyme called *aromatase,* which transforms testosterone into estradiol (a form of estrogen). Preservation of higher testosterone levels may be one reason for damiana's pro-libido effects in both men and women.

Damiana also has anti-anxiety properties that support its use as an aphrodisiac (anxiety works against arousal and desire). Some sources say it has a mild euphoric effect—it's actually an ingredient in some Mexican liqueurs.

Recommendations
Use damiana either in a combination formula or as a tea. If you choose to use the tea, find an organic brand and sip a cup a day.

Precautions
Diabetics should not use damiana because it can affect blood sugar levels, making management of the disease more difficult. It's also not recommended for people who have Parkinson's disease or Alzheimer's disease.

Epimedium (horny goat weed)
This Chinese aphrodisiac is prescribed by herbalists to treat erectile dysfunction, fatigue and menopause symptoms. Its most important use is in reviving sexual vitality for both men and women. Animal studies show that horny goat weed (which supposedly was discovered when a goat herder noticed his goats mating more after grazing on the plant) enhances genital blood flow. It inhibits the same enzyme inhibited by drugs like Viagra, which in turn increases nitric oxide levels in the clitoris or penis. Researchers at the University of California in San Francisco also found that epimedium promotes growth of nerve cells in the pelvic region in rats. Some studies also show a libido-enhancing effect on hormone balance.

Recommendations

Use a supplement that is standardized to 10 percent icariin, which is believed to be the active part of the herb. Use according to the directions on the package.

Precautions

When taken in moderation according to standard guidelines, horny goat weed is very safe.

Ginkgo biloba

The Chinese have used the leaves of the ginkgo tree as a medicine for thousands of years, and it's been a popular herb in North America and Europe for decades. Ginkgo promotes better circulation throughout the body and enhances alertness and energy. These effects are due to ginkgo's influence on nitric oxide levels and the fact that it relaxes smooth muscle (the muscles in the body that aren't consciously controlled, like those that clamp down in the walls of arteries to raise blood pressure and restrict circulation). Ginkgo also has antioxidant effects and improves response to stress in both brain and body.

Ginkgo is especially helpful for reviving libido in people who've lost it as a side effect of antidepressant drug therapy. Women on antidepressants seem to benefit more from ginkgo than men when it's used to relieve this very common side effect—and at least one study found that it improves all four phases of the sexual response cycle (desire, arousal, orgasm and 'afterglow').

Recommendations

Take up to 200 mg of ginkgo biloba leaf per day. Many studies have used a form of ginkgo called EGb 761, which is standardized to contain 24 percent ginkgo-flavonol glycosides and 6 percent terpene lactones. All this means is that every dose of this supplement will contain all the right ingredients to have the positive effects seen in research studies.

Precautions

Ginkgo's side effects can include digestive problems, headaches and a stimulant effect (stimulant as in caffeine, not as in sexual). These side effects often disappear within a few days or weeks.

People who take anticonvulsant medications for epilepsy should know that ginkgo can reduce the effectiveness of those medications.

If you decide to take ginkgo and you are taking a selective serotonin reuptake inhibitor (SSRI) antidepressant, check in with your doctor and pharmacist about switching to a different medication. In combination with high doses of ginkgo, SSRIs can cause serotonin levels to rise too high—a condition called *serotonin syndrome*. This can lead to body stiffness, fast heart rate, low body temperature and sweating. If this ever happens while you are taking an SSRI and ginkgo, see a physician right away.

Ginkgo has a blood pressure-lowering effect. If you take drugs for high blood pressure, monitor blood pressure to make sure it doesn't go too low. You may need to reduce your medication dosage.

If you take any blood thinning drug (like aspirin, Plavix, heparin, Ticlid or Coumadin), do not use ginkgo because it also thins the blood. This could be dangerous if you have a stroke or an injury because your blood may not clot properly. Don't take ginkgo if you are taking a non-steroidal anti-inflammatory drug like ibuprofen, as there has been a report of bleeding in the brain with this combination.

Ginkgo can affect blood sugar levels. If you are diabetic, consult with your health care team before trying ginkgo.

Ginseng

Eleven species of ginseng grow around the world. A few are used as herbal medicines, mainly because of their *adaptogenic* effects. Adaptogens modulate and balance the body's systems, revving up systems that aren't working at their best and soothing systems that are overtaxed or overstimulated. In traditional Chinese medicine, ginseng is included in many herbal formulas prescribed for sexual dysfunction.

Studies show that ginseng enhances nitric oxide levels in the genitals and in the blood vessels that feed the pituitary gland—the "master gland" that regulates libido-producing hormones. It also affects the nervous system, altering levels of body chemicals that bring on feelings of desire. Ginseng is used for its blood pressure-lowering and generally energizing effects. Ginsenosides—its active constituents—also have antioxidant and anti-cancer effects.

Recommendations

Try either American ginseng *(Panax quinquefolium)* or Chinese ginseng *(Panax ginseng)*. So-called Siberian ginseng *(Eleutherococcus senticosus)* is not a real ginseng. Try 100 to 200 mg daily of ginseng standardized to 4 to 7 percent ginsenosides. Many studies have used a form of ginseng called Ginsana (G115), which is standardized to 4 percent ginsenosides.

Precautions

Ginseng may affect your ability to fall asleep; reduce the dose or take it early in the day if this happens.

Because of its mild estrogenic effects, ginseng should be avoided if you have endometriosis, fibroids or an estrogen-sensitive cancer like breast, uterine or ovarian cancer.

Ginseng can enhance the effect of blood thinners such as Ticlid, Coumadin, heparin or aspirin, which could lead to uncontrolled bleeding.

Ginseng's stimulant effects can raise heart rate and blood pressure. If you tend toward high blood pressure, monitor your BP to make sure it stays within healthy limits while using ginseng.

If you take theophylline or albuterol for asthma, ginseng may increase the side effects you experience.

Ginseng can help type 2 diabetics to better manage their blood sugar levels, but (Chinese or Korean) ginseng may impact the effect of drugs like Glucophage, Glynase, Amaryl and Glucotrol XL. Monitor blood sugar closely when starting ginseng to see whether medication doses should be changed.

Ginseng can interact with the antidepressants Nardil and Marplan and the antipsychotic drugs Thorazine and Prolixin.

Maca

Maca is a root vegetable that naturally grows at high altitude in the Peruvian Andes. It has been used as a medicinal food for thousands of years. Like ginseng, it is considered an adaptogen. Modern research supports maca's traditional uses as a libido enhancer and overall energizer. Maca can be used in the form of powder, pill, liquid extract or flour.

As a food, maca has high concentrations of vitamins, minerals, protein and healthy fats. It also contains natural chemicals that impact energy, mood and libido. In studies where men with erectile dysfunction and postmenopausal women were given maca or a placebo, maca promoted strength, endurance, well-being and sexual desire. Some studies have found that maca has a balancing effect on hormones. Other research suggests that this herb can help curb depression and revive libido in people who take antidepressants.

Recommendations

The usual dose of maca is between 1.5 and 3.0 grams (1,500 to 3,000 mg) per day. This would be the dose with maca supplements that are simply ground-up maca root or maca flour encased in a capsule or sold as powder or tablets—basically, the whole food put into supplement form. Some supplements are much more concentrated. Whichever variety of maca you choose, follow the directions on the container.

Precautions

No harmful side effects have been identified even with very high doses of maca, although taking too much could make you jittery.

Maca isn't a good choice for people who have thyroid disease. It contains glucosinolates, which interact with the thyroid gland and can cause goiter in susceptible people who don't get enough iodine in their diets.

Muira Puama (ptychopetalum olacoides) and Catuaba (trichilia catigua)

This pair of herbs from the Amazon rainforest are commonly used to enhance libido in that part of the world. In cities in the Amazon, smoothies with a heaping teaspoon each of muira puama and catuaba are popular evening cocktails said to enhance desire and sexual pleasure.

Both herbs—which are taken from the roots and bark of two Amazonian trees—have antidepressant, anti-anxiety and stress-reducing effects. Muira puama is soothing and relaxing; catuaba is more stimulating. Most of the research on these herbs suggests that they work by increasing levels of the neurotransmitter dopamine, which has a strong libido-boosting effect.

Recommendations

An effective dose of muira puama is about 1.5 grams. It can be taken as a tea, which is brewed strong and sipped once a day. Five hundred milligrams of catuaba a few times weekly can be a good complement to muira puama, but they don't need to be taken together. Many libido-enhancing herbal combinations include one or both of these herbs.

Precautions

When taken according to directions, these herbs are very safe.

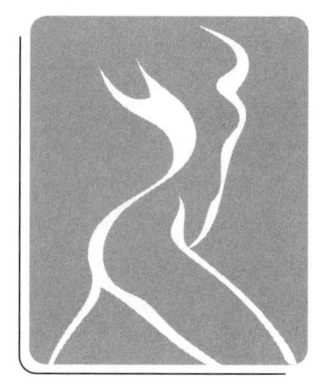

Drugs That Sabotage
Your Sex Life

L ana, a woman in her 40s, came to me with common premenopausal
complaints: breast tenderness, bloating, difficult periods, low libido
and a general feeling of brain fog. She had gained 15 pounds in the
months before coming to see me, but had made no changes in her diet.

"One thing that has helped me get through all this is the medication my
other doctor prescribed," she told me. "I was in a bad mood all the time,
snapping at my family, my friends, my co-workers…I was impossible!
And I was so tired, too…tired *and* hyper, at the same time. It was such a
relief to hear that I wasn't going crazy—it was just depression. The Zoloft
really helped."

As we discussed this further, some troubling information emerged. Sure,
Lana had fewer "downs," but she also didn't have many "ups." She was in

control, but she couldn't seem to get herself to care about much of anything, either. She felt *flat*. And while the Zoloft had helped her moods, it hadn't helped any of her other symptoms. "You probably have deficient amounts of progesterone and testosterone, and it's likely that you have an imbalance of estrogen and progesterone," I told her. "But you don't have a Zoloft deficiency!"

Lana's libido had not been much of an issue until she had started the Zoloft. This came as no surprise to me; as you'll learn in this chapter, most of the people who take drugs in that class have some kind of adverse effect involving sexual desire or sexual function. Fortunately she didn't need to continue on the Zoloft once her hormones and lifestyle were better balanced.

Americans tend to have a strong "pill for every ill" mindset. Drug ads are everywhere, in all media, touting the raising of awareness about this or that newly discovered disorder or the next new miracle medicine. Half of Americans take at least one prescription drug every day. One in every six Americans takes three or more medicines daily—as do five out of every six people over the age of 65. That's a lot of pharmaceuticals being made, marketed, prescribed, bought and used.

This chapter is about the 200+ of these medications that can have a negative impact on libido and sexual function. Sometimes, as in Lana's case, these medications aren't really necessary—they're prescribed to treat a symptom, but don't address the underlying issues that will actually bring healing. Once those issues are addressed, the drug is no longer needed.

Some drugs impact libido or sexual function in many of the people who use them. Others have this effect very rarely. But if a woman has experienced a big drop in libido and is taking one or more medications that may affect sex drive, ability to have orgasm, or ability to enjoy sex—even if the likelihood of this is low—it's important for her to be aware of these possible side effects. She may be able to switch to a different medication that won't affect her sex life, or she may be able, through some simple lifestyle changes or natural remedies, to stop taking the medication altogether.

This being said, let me be clear that some medications are necessary for some people. If you decide to stop or reduce the dose of a prescription medication, please do that under the guidance of a health care professional.

The major classes of medication that affect libido are:

- Hormonal contraception (e.g. birth control pills, patches and Mirena IUD)
- Synthetic hormone replacement medications (e.g. PremPro)
- Psychiatric drugs—those prescribed for depression, anxiety, bipolar disorder, obsessive-compulsive disorder, ADHD and schizophrenia
- Anti-seizure drugs, which are sometimes used to treat bipolar disorder and other psychiatric conditions
- Antihypertensives—drugs that lower blood pressure
- Cholesterol-lowering drugs
- Sleep drugs
- Pain drugs
- Drugs used to treat Parkinson's disease
- Drugs used to manage and treat human immunodeficiency virus (HIV)
- Drugs that ablate (block) hormone production or action, which are used to treat severe hormone-related conditions such as cancers or endometriosis

Sometimes, two similar drugs in the same drug class will have different effects on an individual person's libido. Simply switching from one to another may be enough to reduce impact on sex drive.

Most of the drug classes above will be covered in more detail in this chapter. You'll learn what is known about how this class of drugs affects body chemistry in ways that affect libido. I'll offer insights about how to naturally treat the conditions for which those drugs are prescribed, which might then help to reduce or eliminate the need for libido-dampening medications.

I'll leave out of the discussion the last three categories: drugs used to treat Parkinson's disease, to block hormone production and to treat and manage HIV/AIDS. These medications are only prescribed when absolutely necessary, and there are no real natural alternatives to them. I also won't cover drugs for schizophrenia, OCD or bipolar disorder in depth because the choices faced by people with these conditions are too difficult to address in adequate detail in this book. I will, however, address some of the legal and illegal recreational drugs sometimes used in misguided attempts to boost libido: alcohol, marijuana and cocaine.

Hormonal Contraceptives

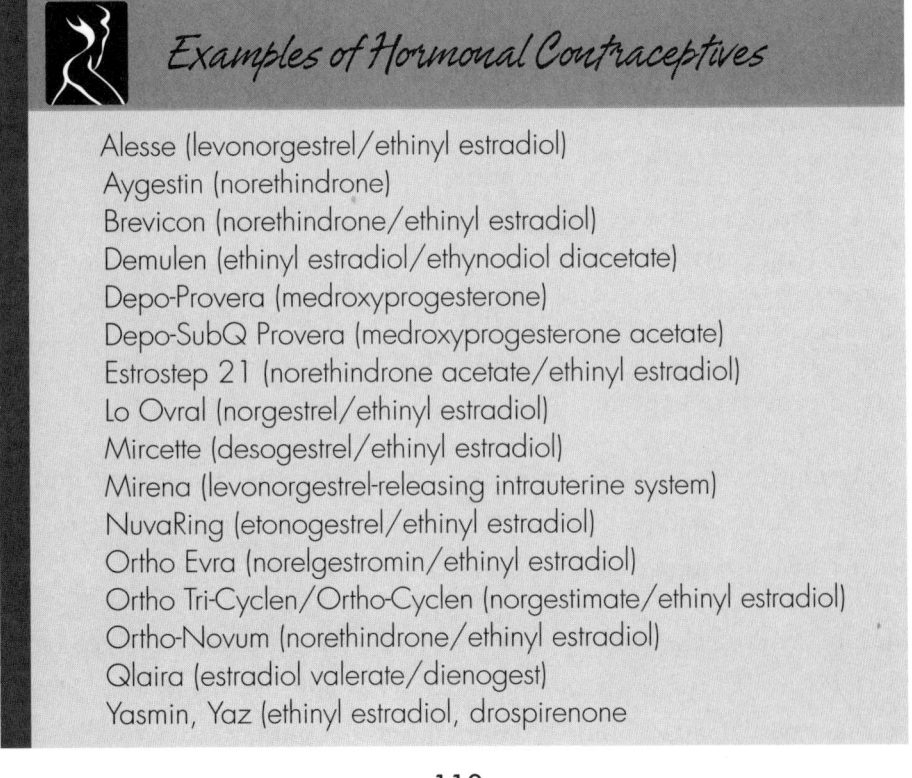

Examples of Hormonal Contraceptives

Alesse (levonorgestrel/ethinyl estradiol)
Aygestin (norethindrone)
Brevicon (norethindrone/ethinyl estradiol)
Demulen (ethinyl estradiol/ethynodiol diacetate)
Depo-Provera (medroxyprogesterone)
Depo-SubQ Provera (medroxyprogesterone acetate)
Estrostep 21 (norethindrone acetate/ethinyl estradiol)
Lo Ovral (norgestrel/ethinyl estradiol)
Mircette (desogestrel/ethinyl estradiol)
Mirena (levonorgestrel-releasing intrauterine system)
NuvaRing (etonogestrel/ethinyl estradiol)
Ortho Evra (norelgestromin/ethinyl estradiol)
Ortho Tri-Cyclen/Ortho-Cyclen (norgestimate/ethinyl estradiol)
Ortho-Novum (norethindrone/ethinyl estradiol)
Qlaira (estradiol valerate/dienogest)
Yasmin, Yaz (ethinyl estradiol, drospirenone

All hormonal contraceptives increase levels of sex hormone-binding glob-ulin, or SHBG. (Estrogens in synthetic hormone replacement [HRT] will also cause SHBG to rise, but the dosages of estrogen from properly prescribed bioidentical HRT are too low to make this a concern.) When SHBG is elevated, more natural testosterone is bound up in it and is no longer active in the body. The "hormone of arousal" gets taken out of play.

In 2006, researchers at Boston University Medical Center conducted a study of women in their 30s with sexual dysfunction. It included 62 wom-en who had been using oral contraceptives (OCs) (the Pill) for more than six months and continued to use them during the course of the study. It also included 39 women who had used OCs for at least six months, then stopped before the study; and included 23 women who had never used OCs. SHBG levels were *four times higher* in the current OC users than in those who had never used OCs.

The most significant part of this study was that the women who had used OCs long term and stopped for up to 120 days continued to have high SHBG levels. They went down, but not to the levels of the women who had never used OCs. This suggests that hormonal contraception might have long-term effects on libido even after the drug is stopped because alterations in SHBG persist.

Hormonal contraception can be delivered through patches, implants, pills, intrauterine devices or IUDs (Mirena), injections or vaginal rings. Synthet-ic hormone replacement (HRT) can be delivered through most of these routes, but the dosages are lower. Most hormonal contraceptives contain both estrogens and progestins—these are known as *combined oral contra-ceptives*, or COCs; others contain only progestins, and they're known as *progestin-only contraceptives* (POPs). COCs and POPs have different side effect profiles: for example, breakthrough bleeding is more common with POPs, while the risk of deep-vein thrombosis (where a blood clot clogs a vein, usually in the lower legs) is more of a concern with COCs.

COCs work by suppressing ovulation. POPs suppress ovulation most of the time but also work by altering cervical mucus in ways that prevent fertilization. In both kinds of hormonal contraception, progestins do the lion's share of the work of un-balancing natural hormone cycles enough to prevent pregnancy from occurring. Knowing what you've learned so far in this book about the importance of normal hormonal cycles in creating libido, it's probably no surprise that these medications can interfere with sex drive.

Combined oral contraceptives are more likely to reduce libido than progestin-only contraceptives. Lower doses of estrogen and progestin will impact libido less than higher doses. When hormones are delivered orally (in pill form), they are more likely to affect libido than they are when delivered by other routes (through skin, intravaginally, through an IUD or by injection). Some progestins have more *androgenic* effects, which means they act a little bit like testosterone; these versions might be recommended by a woman's doctor if she complains of lost libido while using hormonal birth control. Tri-phasics (which contain three different progestin strengths per cycle) are less likely to reduce libido than bi-phasics (with two different progestin strengths per cycle). At any dose, in any schedule, progestins can and do reduce testosterone activity and libido.

Most hormonal contraceptives include a week where no hormone is taken so that the uterine lining can be shed, creating some facsimile of a normal menstrual period. In others, instead of monthly breaks for menstruation, the pills create only four periods per year. This practice of menstrual suppression may be helpful for women with endometriosis or other serious problems, but for others, I don't recommend it. Constant exposure to synthetic hormones month after month—which suppresses the production of natural ovarian hormones with no break—can affect bone health, fertility, and risk of breast cancer, strokes and blood clots. We just don't know whether menstrual suppression is safe—and if it's only being done for convenience, the risks don't balance the benefits.

Overall, I advise women to avoid hormonal contraceptives whether they're given continuously or with breaks once a month. This includes Qlaira, a newer birth control pill that has been marketed as "body-identical." Qlaira does contain a *nearly* bioidentical estrogen… but it also contains very *non-bioidentical* progestins. At this writing, no hormonal contraceptive is truly bioidentical. I recommend barrier methods or a Paragard IUD (the kind that doesn't contain progestins). If you don't plan to become pregnant in the future, look into tubal ligation or a vasectomy for your partner.

Examples of Hormone Replacement Therapy

Note: estradiol is a bioidentical estrogen

Alora (estradiol patch)
Enjuvia (conjugated estrogens)
Cenestin (conjugated estrogens)
Activella (estradiol/norethindrone acetate)
Climara Pro (estradiol, levonorgestrel transdermal)
CombiPatch (estradiol/norethindrone acetate patch)
Delestrogen (estradiol valerate)
Dienestrol (intravaginal synthetic estrogens)
Estrace Vaginal Cream (estradiol vaginal cream)
Estraderm (estradiol patch)
Esclim (estradiol patch)
Estratest (esterified estrogens and methyltestosterone)
Estring (estradiol vaginal ring; also sold as Femring)
EstroGel (estradiol gel)
FemHRT (norethindrone acetate/ethinyl estradiol)
Menest (esterified estrogens, primarily estrone and equilin or horse estrogen)
Angeliq (drospirenone/estradiol)
Ogen (estropipate)
Prefest (estradiol/norgestimate)

Premarin (conjugated estrogens)
Prempro (conjugated estrogens, medroxyprogesterone
    acetate; also sold as Premphase)
Vivelle (estradiol patch)

The way to tell the difference between synthetic and bioidentical hormones in HRT is this: if is just says estradiol, estrone, estriol, progesterone or testosterone, it's bioidentical. If it's conjugated or esterified or has the words ethinyl, methyl, medroxy, etc. in front of it, it's not bioidentical. If it just says "estrogens," it's probably not bioidentical.

HRT contains less progestin and estrogen than hormonal contraceptives. These drugs can still have negative effects on libido. Estrogens in synthetic HRT will help to reverse vaginal atrophy and promote better lubrication, but they can also reduce testosterone activity in the body. Synthetic estrogens create more toxicity because they are processed differently in the body than bioidentical versions.

If you do decide to use HRT, topically applied versions (patches, vaginal rings, creams) are less likely to have a negative impact on libido. When hormones are needed to achieve balance, an individually tailored bioidentical HRT plan that includes testosterone, along with the lifestyle shifts and other recommendations described in this book, will more effectively promote restored libido and sexual sensation.

Hypertension Drugs and Heart Drugs

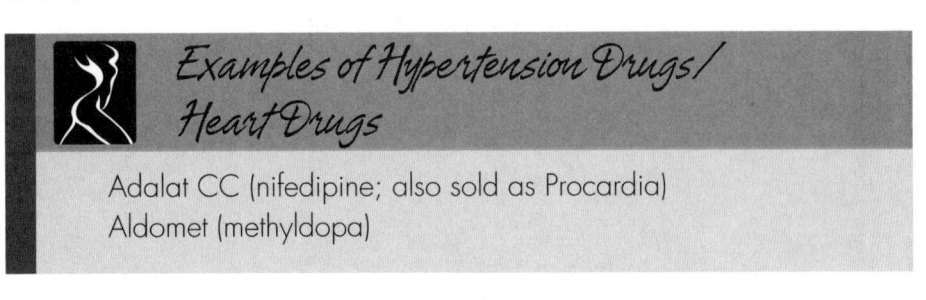

Examples of Hypertension Drugs/ Heart Drugs

Adalat CC (nifedipine; also sold as Procardia)
Aldomet (methyldopa)

Aldoril (methyldopa/hydrochlorothiazide)
Avalide (irbesartan/hydrochlorothiazide)
Avapro (irbesartan)
Blocadren (timolol)
Caduet (amodipine besylate/atorvastatin calcium)
Catapres (clonidine)
Clorpres (clonidine hydrochloride and chlorthalidone)
Cordarone (amiodarone HCl)
Coreg (carvedilol)
Corgard (nadolol)
Corzide (nadolol/bendroflumethiazide)
Cosopt (dorzolamide hydrochloride/timolol maleate)
Cardura (doxazosin mesylate)
Cozaar (losartan potassium)
Diovan HCT (valsartan/hydrochlorothiazide)
Dynacirc (isradipine)
Guanfacine hydrochloride (guanfacine)
Hyzaar (losartan potassium/hydrochlorothiazide)
Inversine (mecamylamine)
Kerlone (betaxolol hydrochloride)
Lescol (fluvastatin sodium)
Lexxel (enalapril maleate/felodipine)
Lopressor (metoprolol tartrate)
Lotensin (benazepril)
Lotensin HCT (benazepril HCl/hydrochlorothiazide)
Lotrel (amlodipine besylate/benazepril HCl)
Lozol (indapamide)
Mavik (trandolapril)
Mexitil (mexiletine HCl)
Midamor (amiloride) HTX
Moduretic (amiloride/hydrochlorothiazide)
Monopril (fosinopril sodium)
Plendil (felodipine)
Prinivil (lisinopril)

Prinzide (lisinopril/hydrochlorothiazide)
Sular (nisoldipine)
Tambocor (flecainide)
Toprol XL (metoprolol succinate)
Vascor (bepridil)
Zebeta (bisoprolol fumarate)
Ziac (bisopropolol/hydrochlorothiazide)

It has long been known that hypertension or high blood pressure—greater than 140/90 mmHg—has a negative impact on a man's ability to get and keep an erection. Untreated hypertension can also impact libido and arousal in women. One in three American adults has blood pressure levels that qualify as hypertensive, and there are many cases of undiagnosed hypertension. If your libido is low and you don't know what your blood pressure is, have it checked to be sure that hypertension isn't contributing to the problem. Unfortunately, many drugs prescribed to reduce blood pressure can also diminish libido.

The reasons for this effect vary depending on whether the drug is a beta blocker (their generic names all end in –lol), a diuretic, a calcium channel blocker or an ACE inhibitor.

Beta-blockers are more likely to affect libido than calcium channel blockers, diuretics or ACE inhibitors. In my practice, I commonly recommend that patients who use beta-blockers get a prescription for an anti-hypertensive drug from a different class.

If you take a medication for high blood pressure and it appears on the list of drugs above—all of which have lowered libido or decreased sexual performance listed in their side effect profiles—talk with your doctor about trying a different medication. Better yet, you may want to consider side-effect-free natural remedies for high blood pressure. (Don't stop taking blood pressure medication on your own. Having out-of-control hypertension is worse for libido than taking any of these medications.)

Everyone's blood pressure rises with age. Kidney disease, hormonal disorders or even some prescription drugs (including oral contraceptives) and herbs (including licorice and ginseng) can cause blood pressure to rise above healthy levels. Being overweight, smoking, drinking excessive amounts of alcohol and lack of exercise all increase risk. Many people have a hereditary tendency to develop hypertension.

To address hypertension naturally, first be sure that medications or herbs aren't responsible. Back off of the alcohol if you have more than one drink per day, and of course quit smoking if you still haven't.

Here are some recommendations for lowering blood pressure naturally:

- Follow the guidelines in Chapter 9 to drop excess weight and eat a nutrient-dense diet that's low in sweets and processed foods.

- Try yoga, biofeedback or *autogenic training* (a way of learning to control blood pressure and other automatic body functions), all of which have been found to help lower blood pressure.

- Take advantage of the recommendations for stress management in Chapter 8.

- Reduce salt intake to below 2,400 milligrams per day—not hard to do once you get processed and packaged foods out of your life. More salt-sensitive people may want to reduce salt even more, to 1,500 mg per day.

- Get some aerobic exercise at least four times a week—preferably, integrate this into your life every day in some way.

- Try supplements with documented blood pressure-lowering effects: coenzyme Q10 (50 to 200 mg per day), and garlic (2 to 4 raw cloves per day, or 300 mg dried garlic in capsule form, or 7.2

grams per day of aged garlic). Follow the guidelines for fish oil, calcium, magnesium and potassium intake given in Chapter 9.

Cholesterol-Lowering Drugs

Examples of Cholesterol-Lowering Drugs

Advicor (niacin XR/lovastatin)
Altoprev (lovastatin extended-release tablets)
Antara (fenofibrate)
Atromid-S (clofibrate)
Zetia (ezetimibe)
Pravachol (pravastatin sodium)
Caduet (amodipine besylate/atorvastatin calcium)
Lipitor (atorvastatin calcium)
Lopid (gemfibrozil)
Lipofen (fenofibrate)
Mevacor (lovastatin)
Questran (cholestyramine)
Zocor (simvastatin)

The statin medications used to reduce cholesterol levels are the world's top-selling drugs. Some 200 million prescriptions for these medicines are written each year to lower cholesterol levels. Older cholesterol-lowering drugs—including fibrates and cholestyramine—are prescribed far less often because they are associated with more side effects.

Most of the research demonstrating the libido-lowering effect of statins are about erectile dysfunction (ED), which is relatively easy to measure: does erection occur and is it maintained long enough to accomplish intercourse? Female sexual arousal and response are more complex and difficult to quantify in a scientific study. But when we look at the reasons why cholesterol-lowering drugs often lead to ED, we can understand the potential for the same effect in women.

Cholesterol is a necessary building block for the hormones of sexual arousal, including testosterone, estrogens and progesterone. Studies of men who lose erectile function while on statins have found that their testosterone levels fall in response to the medication, and that testosterone rises again when the drug is stopped. Another effect of blocking cholesterol production with statins is reduced production of a nutrient called *coenzyme Q10* (CoQ10), which plays a role in producing energy at the cellular level and in providing energy to muscles. CoQ10 depletion has been linked to many of the side effects of statin drugs, including increased risk of heart failure, muscle pain and intense fatigue. If you feel exhausted and achy, renewing your love life is bound to fall off of your short list of concerns.

In general, doctors will tell you that statin drugs reduce the risk of a first heart attack or stroke when prescribed to treat high levels of LDL (low-density lipoprotein) cholesterol, the "bad" cholesterol that has been linked to heart disease. However, in studies, this protective effect has only been shown for people between the ages of 55 and 65 who have already suffered a heart attack or stroke. Furthermore, the protective effect in this group is more significant for men than for women.

It isn't even completely clear *how* statins are protective. They do lower cholesterol, but they also have anti-inflammatory effects—and with what's known now about the role of inflammation in cardiovascular disease, this effect may turn out to be even more important than that of lowering cholesterol.

What most doctors won't tell you about statins is that they have a long laundry list of side effects. People taking statins can suffer from mental fogginess, weakness, depression and muscle pain. Some statin users experience severe cognitive impairment or *transient global amnesia* (TGA)—an episode where there's total memory loss for a short period of time. If lowered libido is also thrown into the mix, a small decrease in risk of cardiovascular disease doesn't seem like such a good tradeoff.

Cholesterol is a necessary and important substance. It's used by the body to build the brain, the nerves and the steroid hormones (including estrogen, progesterone, testosterone, DHEA and cortisol) and is needed to make vitamin D. Good immune function and digestion of fat-soluble nutrients such as vitamins E and vitamin A also depend on adequate stores of cholesterol. Cholesterol is so important that we get only one quarter of it through diet; the rest is made in the liver. The body efficiently decreases its own production of cholesterol when more comes in through the diet. This is why eating a diet with little or no cholesterol has minimal effect on cholesterol counts.

If your total cholesterol is over 200 or your LDL is over 130, you are likely to end up with a prescription for a cholesterol-lowering drug, especially if you have other risk factors for cardiovascular disease, which include obesity, high triglycerides (a type of blood fat), high blood pressure, and diabetes. (Many experts believe that if you don't have other risk factors, it's okay to say "no thanks" to cholesterol lowering even if your numbers are a bit high—but you'll likely be advised to alter your diet or use other natural methods to try to bring LDL down and HDL up.)

If you are taking a statin and suspect that this might be affecting your libido, here are some strategies for reducing cholesterol naturally. These interventions will also reduce inflammation and help rein in other cardiovascular disease risk factors.

How to reduce cholesterol without drugs

- Take psyllium, a type of supplemental fiber. The insoluble fiber in psyllium helps the body to eliminate more cholesterol. In one study, supplementing with psyllium for eight weeks lowered LDL, triglycerides, insulin and blood pressure and raised HDL. Take a half teaspoon of psyllium in eight ounces of water two to three times a day. (Drink immediately after adding the fiber, before the psyllium thickens.)

- The diet recommended in Chapter 9 with particular attention to reducing sugar and refined carbohydrates, exercise, garlic and fish oil all help to reduce LDL and raise HDL.

- Green tea lowers cholesterol. Try sipping green tea two or three times a day or take a supplement that contains green tea catechins. Follow the directions on the container.

- Artichoke leaf extract has been found to lower LDL and raise HDL. Try 1,800 to 1,920 mg per day, divided into two to three doses.

Psychiatric Drugs, Sleep Drugs, and Anti-Seizure Drugs

Examples of Psychiatric Drugs, Sleep Drugs and Anti-Seizure Drugs

Abilify (aripiprazole)
Amoxapine AD
Ambien CR (zolpidem tartrate)
Anafranil (clomipramine HCl)
Ativan (lorazepam)
Buspar (buspirone) antianxiety
Celexa (citalopram hydrobromate)
Clozaril (clozapine)
Concerta (methylphenidate)
Desoxyn (methamphetamine hydrochloride)
Dexedrine (dextroamphetamine)
Effexor (venlafaxine hydrochloride)

Elavil (amitryptiline)
Emsam (selegiline)
Fazaclo (clozapine)
Gabitril (tiagabine HCl)
Haldol (haloperidol)
Klonopin (clonazepam)
Lamictal (lamortrigine)
Lexapro (escitalopram oxalate)
Librium (chlordiazepoxide)
Lunesta (eszopiclone)
Luvox (fluvoxamine maleate)
Mirapex (pramipexole)
Moban (molindone hydrochloride)
Norpramin (desipramine hydrochloride)
Pamelor (nortriptyline HCl)
Paxil (paroxetine; also sold as Paxil-CR, Pexeva, Asimia)
Perphenazine
Prolixin (fluphenazine)
Prosom (estazolam)
Prozac (fluoxetine)
Remeron (mirtazapine)
Risperdal (risperidone)
Serax (oxazepam)
Seroquel (quetiapine fumarate)
Serzone (nefazodone)
Sinequan (doxepin)
Tofranil (imipramine)
Trileptal (oxcarbazepine)
Valium (diazepam)
Xanax (alprazolam; also sold as Niravam)
Zarontin (ethosuximide)
Zoloft (sertraline)
Zyban (bupropion HCl)
Zyprexa (olanzapine)

Many of the drugs prescribed for depression, anxiety, bipolar disorder, obsessive-compulsive disorder, insomnia, ADHD, schizophrenia and other psychiatric diagnoses affect libido. The same goes for some anti-seizure drugs, which are prescribed for epilepsy, and for depression, bipolar disorder and other psychological disorders that don't respond well to milder medications.

Neurotransmitters, which are the body chemicals that are 'tweaked' by psychiatric drugs, play an important but not well understood role in orchestrating libido. When we tinker with neurotransmitter balance with medications, libido can be strongly impacted. Orgasms can become difficult to achieve for people taking many of the medicines listed above, and some report that the orgasms they do have are pleasureless. Genitals can become numb on many of these medicines. For most women, healthy libido requires ready access to emotions; this can be blunted by medications given to treat depression, anxiety and other psychiatric diagnoses.

Selective serotonin-reuptake inhibitors (SSRIs) such as Zoloft, Prozac, Celexa, Lexapro, Luvox, Paxil, Lustral and Sarafem cause sexual side effects in roughly 40 percent of the people who take them. Some research even suggests that this number should be as high as 80 percent. The SNRIs, a related class of drugs that include Cymbalta and Effexor, affect two neurotransmitters (serotonin and norepinephrine) and are believed to have similarly high rates of sexual side effects. A few reports suggest that in some people, sexual dysfunction caused by psychiatric drugs persists even after the drug is discontinued. Drugs for ADHD, bipolar disorder, anxiety and OCD all affect neurotransmitters and have sexual side effects.

This is not to say that if you have a serious mental disorder, you should stop your medications cold turkey to save your libido or your sexual function. Epileptics, people with severe bipolar or obsessive-compulsive disease, or those who get too anxious or depressed to function for long periods of time may have to stay on medication. If this describes you, discuss medication options with your doctor and pharmacist to see whether your medicines can be shifted or dosages changed in order to help you reclaim your sex life.

In my opinion, antidepressants, anti-anxiety drugs, sleep drugs and ADHD drugs are being prescribed to large numbers of people who do not really need them! Feeling blue, tired or overwhelmed isn't reason enough to pharmacologically tamper with your neurotransmitters. Therapy, stress management, regular exercise and good nutrition may be all you need to wean yourself off these libido-sapping medications.

Drugs that help people get to sleep and stay asleep—such as Ambien, Lunesta, Halcion, Rozerem and Prosom—cost Americans over $4.5 billion per year. They work through the same mechanism as anti-anxiety drugs. Although people who take them tend to think they're helping a lot, research has demonstrated that subjects with insomnia only get about 25 minutes of additional sleep compared to those who take an inert placebo pill!

Nobody should stop taking an antidepressant, antipsychotic or anti-seizure drug suddenly—all of these types of medication need to be tapered over time with medical support. Withdrawal symptoms can be difficult, and in rare cases, severe. Tampering with your dosages without medical support is never a good idea.

There are supplements that can help relieve depression and anxiety and promote better sleep, and hormone balancing often relieves these symptoms.

Remedies for depression:

- Fish oil, taken in slightly higher doses than recommended in Chapter 9, shows promise in helping people with symptoms of anxiety, mild depression, bipolar disorder and ADHD. To experiment with this, increase your dose of fish oil to three grams of DHA/EPA per day.

- St. John's wort is an herb that gently shifts neurotransmitters in a way similar to that of SSRIs with fewer side effects. Try 300 to 1,800 mg a day. **Be sure not to use St. John's wort with any psychiatric medication or with SAM-e (see below) or 5-HTP (also described below).** Combining agents that raise serotonin levels can cause serotonin syndrome, which is a serious problem. Allow three weeks between stopping an SSRI or SNRI and starting St. John's wort.

- S-adenosylmethionine (SAM-e) has been used in Europe as a prescription drug for depression since the mid-1980s. Like St. John's wort, it affects neurotransmitter levels gently. SAM-e isn't a good choice for anxiety or for those with manic tendencies because it has stimulant properties. Try 200 mg twice a day for a few days, then increase to 400 mg twice a day. **Don't use with psychiatric medications, St. John's wort or 5-HTP.**

- 5-hydroxytryptophan (5-HTP) is a precursor (chemical building block) for serotonin and can be used as a natural remedy for anxiety or depression. Take 150 to 300 mg per day. **Don't use with any psychiatric medication or with SAM-e or St. John's wort.**

Remedies for anxiety or sleeplessness:

- The herbs valerian and passionflower have been used for centuries as natural relaxants. Before turning to libido-sapping prescription drugs, try anti-anxiety teas or herbal supplements.

- If you tend to be anxious, yoga, meditation, breathing exercises, spiritual practices and mindfulness are far superior to medications as antidotes. A good therapist should also be able to help you reduce anxiety that doesn't respond to these other interventions.

- A vigorous, sweaty workout can do wonders for anxiety.

- Often, anxiety comes from thought patterns or ways of living our lives that are inefficient or self-defeating. Seek out therapy or coaching to help change patterns that create difficulty. For example: women often have difficulty clearly asking for what they need, and they then end up feeling anxious and frustrated because their needs aren't being met! It takes practice to be able to ask for what you really need when you're used to ignoring your own needs in order to take care of others. Good therapy or coaching can help with this.

- Melatonin is a hormone made in the pineal gland, which is located in the brain just behind the center of the forehead. Supplemental melatonin makes a great sleep aid for the occasional bout of insomnia or to readjust your inner clock when you've switched time zones. Don't use it every night, as it may cause your pineal gland to get a little lazy and produce less melatonin on its own. Take 0.5 to 2 mg in a sublingual tablet, which dissolves under the tongue and acts quickly. To promote better melatonin production, keep your home lighting minimal after sunset, and have your bedroom as dark as possible when you go to bed (even an LED clock can substantially reduce melatonin production).

- Try taking a combination of 600 mg calcium and 300 mg magnesium just before bed.

Self-Medication: Alcohol, Marijuana and Cocaine

Research has shown that while alcohol might help some women shed inhibitions and feel sexy, it often impedes sexual arousal, delays orgasm, and can even make orgasm impossible to reach. Women who drink too much often report that they feel more aroused, but the mechanisms of arousal—

increased blood flow to the vulva and vagina and lubrication—are reduced following alcohol consumption.

In a laboratory study, 18 women masturbated while having vaginal blood flow and length of time to orgasm measured. They were given varying amounts of alcohol. Women whose blood alcohol levels went up but stayed below the legal limit for driving had lower measurements of sexual arousal. Orgasm was delayed and less intense than for those who had not had any alcohol. At the same time that these physical results were recorded, the women reported that they felt *more* aroused and had more pleasurable orgasms with alcohol than without!

Why these contradictory results? Remember that for women, the *subjective* experience of sex often doesn't seem to match the measurable aspects of it: length of time to orgasm, vaginal or clitoral blood flow, and lubrication. These differences are in the mind. They're about attention, awareness, expectations, thoughts and emotions. It may be that women expect to have a better time in bed when they've had a drink or two, and so they do. Or it may be that loss of inhibition helps women to feel more attractive, more attracted and freer to ask for what they really want during sex.

It's interesting to note that while a drink or two appears to reduce testosterone production in men, the same amount of alcohol appears to *enhance* testosterone production in premenopausal women. Testosterone levels don't appear to be affected by alcohol in women who are past menopause, but alcohol does seem to impact estrogens in postmenopausal women. Those who consume over 25 grams of alcohol (just under one ounce, roughly the amount in a single drink) per day have higher levels of more powerful estrogens (estrone, estradiol) than postmenopausal women who drink moderately or not at all. This may be one reason why women who drink more alcohol are at higher risk of breast cancer.

Yes, alcohol can help loosen you up and get you in the mood, but overconsumption is likely to reduce libido and performance, and could increase breast cancer risk over the long haul. Limit alcohol consumption to one beer or glass of wine a few days a week.

Although marijuana can help loosen inhibitions and alter consciousness in ways that can enhance sexual experience, it reduces testosterone levels in both men and women. Men who smoke a lot of marijuana tend to lose interest in sex. Cocaine can also work as a sex enhancer, but the almost inevitable spiral of addiction and abuse is, obviously, not going to improve your sex life—and it'll probably ruin the rest of your life as well. For men, cocaine has the paradoxical effect of increasing desire but reducing erectile function. This drug carries other big risks, such as heart attack and organ failure.

Mindfulness, breathwork and other tips and tricks recommended in Chapter 8 work just as well as drugs or alcohol for achieving a relaxed state of awareness and heightened sensation.

Knowing Your Options

Only you, with the support of your family and your medical team, can know whether you really need a medication or not. If your libido and your sex life are important to you, you can find ways to enrich it and make it work even if you have to take a medication.

Deciding to stop taking a drug may entail making big shifts in lifestyle, diet, exercise habits or other habits. For some, certain medicines are indispensable. Other medicines are almost never really necessary and tend to be prescribed because doctors aren't aware of other options, or believe patients won't make the necessary lifestyle changes.

Don't just accept the "pill-for-every-ill" mindset. Do your homework and know your options. Your sex life is worth it.

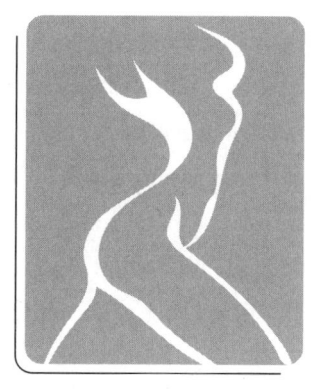

CHAPTER 8

How to Resolve Stress and Fatigue and Increase Libido with Lifestyle Changes

Monica is a 44-year-old mother of three children. She and her husband both work full time running their own small business. While the kids are at school, she keeps the company's books, answers the phone, and keeps the office going while her husband manages employees. With the economic downturn, their business is suffering, and Monica sees that they will either have to lay off several employees or stop offering health insurance. Even keeping up with their household bills is a challenge these days.

By 3 p.m., Monica is playing chauffeur, tutor and referee: driving the children to their after-school activities, helping with homework in waiting areas at the ballet school and the ice rink, and breaking up fights between siblings in the car as they zoom around town.

When they get home, Monica tosses a couple of frozen pizzas in the oven and has her 14-year-old make a salad. They eat in a rush so the children can bathe and finish their homework in time for bed. After bedtime, she and her husband spend an hour tidying the house, folding laundry and putting it away, and checking their personal email accounts, which are full of events to schedule and places to be. As she notices how stiff her body feels, she chides herself for having gone yet another day without a workout.

By 11 p.m. she's "tired but wired," trying to unwind in front of the TV. When her husband comes to her with an amorous look in his eye, it's not hard to guess what she says to him. It's the same thing she says nine times out of every ten times he suggests that they have sex.

Monica's stress level is high even without other common problems such as marital problems, difficult co-workers, unemployment, children who are having serious problems at school or at home, ill parents to care for or health problems. Add any of these issues, and Monica's burden of stress could become even worse. Her husband, as kind and helpful as he is, is not likely to get the sex he wants as long as her current schedule, lack of sleep and levels of worry continue. As for Monica, she misses the romance and pleasure of sex, but she's too wrung out to go there.

Fatigue is the single biggest complaint I hear from my patients—especially those who have lost their libido. I'm happy to say that, thanks to my training in preventive medicine, I'm able to help the majority of my patients regain their energy. Once energy is restored, we can balance hormones and work on the libido.

Stress Douses the Fires of Libido

Whether the body is faced with concerns that are truly dangerous (some kind of immediate threat to safety, for example) or with less urgent, chronic stresses (the kind faced by Monica), it launches what's known as the *stress response*. Much of this response is created by hormones produced by the *adrenals*, two walnut-sized glands that sit just above the kidneys.

When we are in a stressful situation, the brain sends signals to the adrenals to produce the "fight or flight" hormones *adrenaline* and *epinephrine*, which are also called *catecholamines*. The catecholamines constrict blood vessels and quicken heartbeat and rate of breathing, which then circulates oxygen more quickly to working muscles. Stored sugars are released into the bloodstream to fuel the muscles in their efforts to fight or flee.

Another hormone, *cortisol*, is produced by the adrenals in response to chronic, long-term stress. Cortisol works against the hormone insulin to keep blood sugar levels higher than they would be in non-stressful situations. Sensitivity to pain is reduced, and some parts of the brain get more alert while others get less so. This is how intense alertness can coexist with mental fogginess—cortisol activates the parts of the brain that respond best during stressful situations but de-activates other parts that are good at thinking, reasoning, remembering and daydreaming.

Combined, all of these stress hormones cause blood flow to the digestive and sexual organs to drop so that more blood can circulate to heart, lungs and muscles. This re-direction of blood flow also reduces circulation to the skin, which makes it harder to achieve the state of relaxed awareness most likely to lead to sexual desire and pleasure.

The human body's stress response is designed for dealing with urgent stresses, not for the kind of chronic, ongoing stress most of us live with. Our stress is more likely to be *psychosocial*—generated by thoughts, concerns, non-life-threatening fears and obligations. The brain, which regulates these hormones, doesn't register a difference between true fight-or-flight stresses and psychosocial stresses. It responds to both in a similar way. When the stress hormones are constantly released over days, weeks, months and years, cortisol levels settle into a "new normal" where they are constantly elevated. Chronically elevated cortisol creates imbalances in the hormones progesterone, estrogen, insulin and thyroid. This perfect storm of hormonal imbalance can cause anxiety, irritability, mood swings, difficulty sleeping and stress-related illnesses such as high blood pressure, type 2 diabetes, headaches and muscle pain.

Dr. David Zava of ZRT Laboratory, and co-author of the book *What Your Doctor May Not Tell you about Breast Cancer*, explains the balance between cortisol and the other hormones:

"Too much cortisol…causes the tissues to no longer respond to the thyroid hormone signal. It creates a condition of thyroid resistance, meaning that thyroid hormone levels can be normal, but tissues fail to respond as efficiently to the thyroid signal. This resistance to the thyroid hormone signal caused by high cortisol is not just restricted to thyroid hormone but applies to all other hormones such as insulin, progesterone, estrogens, testosterone, and even cortisol itself. When cortisol gets too high, you start getting resistance from the hormone receptors, and it requires more hormones to create the same effect. That's why chronic stress, which elevates cortisol levels, makes you feel so rotten—none of the hormones are allowed to work at optimal levels.

"Insulin resistance is a classic example. It takes more insulin to drive glucose into the cells when cortisol is high. High cortisol and high insulin, resulting in insulin resistance, are going to cause you to gain weight around the waist because your body will store fat there rather than burn it."

High cortisol leads to high insulin levels, which causes more fat to be stored in the body, particularly in the belly area. Chronic stress may play a role in causing heart disease and some cancers. It can reduce immunity, making us more susceptible to colds, flu and other contagious diseases, and may worsen asthma. Although some people do seem more biologically prone to developing anxiety disorders and depressive disorders, these common psychological diagnoses can be triggered or worsened by unrelenting stress. It's estimated that at least two-thirds of doctor visits in the U.S. are due to stress-related complaints.

How would you know whether the stress you're experiencing is causing depleted adrenals? If you're gaining a lot of weight around your midsection without any changes in your diet; if you crave sugar and get shaky between meals; if your skin seems thin or papery; if you're experiencing memory loss; and if your muscles seem to be wasting away, you may have chronically high cortisol levels. Do you get that afternoon low, where all you want to do it lie down and take a nap? It may be your adrenals asking for a break.

Eventually, the adrenals can become exhausted because they are no longer able to keep up with the body's demand for catecholamines and cortisol. This is *adrenal insufficiency*, or *adrenal exhaustion*. Although adrenal insufficiency is not a common diagnosis among conventional medical doctors, those who practice integrative and preventive medicine know it to be epidemic among working mothers. (It gets misdiagnosed as many other things in mainstream medical practices, including depression, and is usually treated with antidepressants and sleeping pills.)

Symptoms of adrenal insufficiency include constant fatigue, muscle weakness, difficulty getting out of bed in the morning even after a good night's sleep, lowered metabolism, and low reserves for coping with stress—even a slight stress beyond the norm creates exhaustion. Other signs of adrenal fatigue: menstrual irregularities, low blood pressure, infertility, poor resistance to urinary tract infections and flu, and depression, which is often caused by all of the other symptoms! It's depressing to be constantly exhausted and depleted.

Women with tired adrenals will have no libido, which is why, once again, one of the sexiest things a man can do is wash the dishes or do a load of laundry. A chronically exhausted woman who is seeking hormonal balance and a restored libido has to begin by normalizing cortisol levels.

Adrenal recovery

Treating adrenal fatigue begins with rest. Adequate sleep, stress management practices, and time for pleasurable activities are the first steps toward renewal.

Most women with stress-caused fatigue have what I call "tired" adrenals. The adrenals aren't exhausted yet but need some help. Creating disciplined sleep habits and making some dietary changes are often enough to restore energy.

For women with tired adrenals, I'll often prescribe adrenal extracts and if needed will add supportive herbs such as ginseng, Ashwagandha and licorice.

Women with tired adrenals often have low blood pressure and crave salty foods—it's healthier to add a little bit of sea salt to a glass of water than to snack on potato chips!

If your adrenals are tired, the last thing in the world you want to do is flog them with sugar, caffeine and other stimulants! See Chapter 9 for guidance on how to establish eating habits that will support the adrenals and the libido.

The sexiness of a good night's sleep

Compounding the stress experienced by many women is lack of sleep. Around 40 percent of people have difficulty sleeping at least some of the time, and 10 percent have chronic insomnia. In a 2010 study by the National Sleep Foundation, 20 percent of adults surveyed stated that they were often too tired for sex. Lack of quality sleep creates even more stress as we try to keep up with our responsibilities while in a wired, tired daze.

Among women, the two most common reasons for sleep loss are young children and menopause.

For parents whose babies are waking up a lot at night or not sleeping through the night after three to five months, I recommend "Ferberizing," a method for teaching babies to fall asleep on their own, popularized by Richard Ferber, M.D. In spite of myths and rumors to the contrary, used properly, the Ferber method is a very gentle and reassuring way to teach babies how to fall asleep on their own, and usually works within a week. It doesn't work for everyone, but for many sleep-deprived parents, it can be a life- and libido-saver.

The hormonal fluctuations that come with menopause can turn a sound sleeper into a wide-eyed tosser and turner. For women who are estrogen dominant, using a progesterone cream or pill before bed can solve their sleep problems literally overnight! Women who are supplementing with testosterone or estrogen should be aware that too much of either can cause insomnia. Adrenal extracts can also causes insomnia, and most people shouldn't take them after 3 p.m.

Of course stress can cause sleeplessness, both because mind chatter keeps us awake and because high cortisol levels can make it nearly impossible to sleep.

Everyone's sleep needs are different. As a general rule, children and teens need more sleep than adults, and older adults need less than younger adults. Six or seven hours of sleep might be plenty for one person, while others do much better with nine hours. Some people thrive when they can take a nap in the afternoon, while others wake up from a nap tired and cranky.

I often recommend that my patients keep a sleep journal for a few weeks in order to track hours of sleep per night and compare that to mood and energy levels. They may find out that on nights they drink alcohol they don't sleep as well and when they've exercised they sleep like a baby. It's amazing how quickly this simple approach can help someone figure out how much sleep they need and why they aren't sleeping.

The bedtime routine should ideally begin an hour before you want to be asleep and might include a hot bath, some gentle stretching and soothing music. Reading a book or watching TV to wind down is OK, as long as there isn't too much excitement or violence involved. (Avoid news shows!) Brew a cup of chamomile or passionflower tea and cuddle up with your partner. Of course sex can be a wonderful sleep aid too! Avoid eating for the last two to three hours before bed and don't consume caffeine after midafternoon. If you're very sensitive to caffeine, don't consume it after late morning.

Don't light up your house like a landing strip until midnight. This will disrupt the body's natural sleep cycles, which are facilitated by a hormone called melatonin. Melatonin is produced by the brain in response to fading light. Once full darkness has fallen outside, allow melatonin production to begin to rise by keeping lights low. Avoid brightly lit computer and TV screens for at least an hour before you want to be asleep.

The bedroom should be dark, quiet and cool at night. Even the brightness from a digital clock can affect sleep by reducing the body's production of melatonin. Cool temperatures in the bedroom will help promote deeper sleep. If the bed is uncomfortable enough to keep you awake, get a new one. Sleep is that important!

If insomnia is an issue for you, try natural sleep aids first. Melatonin supplements often help in falling asleep and staying asleep. If you have trouble falling asleep, get a sublingual brand that dissolves under the tongue and take it a half-hour before bed. If you have trouble staying asleep, try an oral extended release form of melatonin. If melatonin isn't helpful, try herbs such as valerian, passionflower and theanine (a relaxant derived from green tea). Use prescription sleep aids only as a last resort; they're addicting and have been linked to some very strange side effects, including sleep eating and sleep *driving*!

Although snoring is more common in men than women, it can cause poor quality sleep and increases the risk of heart disease and stroke. If you're getting feedback that you snore, take the steps recommended below. Snoring husbands can be serious sleep-robbers. Have him sleep on his side; if he keeps rolling onto his back, try the tennis ball trick (before bed, put a tennis ball on his back and hold it in place with an ACE bandage). Obesity is a major cause of snoring. Some snorers benefit from nasal strips that hold the nasal passages open. Others snore less when they avoid alcohol or dairy products. If snoring is persistent and loud, you or your partner should be checked for sleep apnea.

With adequate rest, the desire to have sex may become stronger than the desire to fall asleep right after dinner.

Mindfulness –
The Ultimate Stress Management

Mindfulness may be the single biggest secret to both a good night's sleep and restoring libido, and I say this with assurance because it has saved my marriage and my sanity. I love my husband, my children and my career, but juggling these roles can be daunting and stressful. By learning how to practice mindfulness, I can manage stress anytime, anywhere, and without any props. To de-stress I don't need a massage, or a cocktail or a pill, I just need to pause long enough to go within, take a deep breath, and refocus on what's important right now.

With mindfulness, we learn how to respond to life's stressors in a way that's healthy and productive. Although mindfulness has its roots in Buddhist practices, it has been successfully used and adapted to Western psychology since the mid-1960s and is a mainstay in the treatment of anxiety disorders, addiction, post-traumatic stress syndrome and depression. Many of my patients have integrated the principles of mindfulness into their own religious and spiritual practices.

When a patient comes to me for help with low libido, I test her hormones and prescribe hormone replacement if needed. I make recommendations about diet, exercise and nutritional supplements. And I suggest that she read Eckhart Tolle's book, *The Power of Now*, or Byron Katie's book, *Loving What Is*.

Tolle draws on wisdom from many spiritual traditions to make the point that the chatter in our heads—not our actual life situations—are the main source of our unhappiness and stress. He writes: "Not to be able to stop thinking is a dreadful affliction, but we don't realize this because almost everybody is suffering from it, so it is considered normal. This incessant mental noise prevents you from finding that realm of inner stillness that is inseparable from Being. It also creates a false mind-made self that casts a shadow of fear and suffering."

Byron Katie offers an elegantly simple approach that she calls "The Work," which involves four questions and a "turnaround." Katie explains that suffering and stress are created when we believe our thoughts and stories. Her four questions are designed to help unravel the truth and bring us to the present moment.

Let's say Monica is driving to a meeting. Her thoughts might go something like this: *I'm gonna be late for the PTA meeting. I HATE being late! I hope the kids are okay. Their dad probably forgot to pick them up. I'm so sick of having to keep track of EVERYTHING for this family. It sucks that I don't have cell reception out here. Oh, crap, I forgot the grocery list. How irresponsible. I'm getting so foggy in my old age. I wish I had one of those fancy blended mochas, but I already ate those chips at lunch today—last thing I need is an 800-calorie coffee drink, with these thighs! Everyone's driving like an idiot…come on, people, it's just a little rain, you can go faster!*

Monica is revving up her stress levels—and her stress hormone levels—with worries, negative statements, exaggerations of her situation, and judgments of herself and others: she's going to be late for a meeting; her husband is forgetful and her kids might have been forgotten; she ought to be able to talk on the phone whenever she wants to; she's irresponsible, foggy, old, and needs to lose weight; everyone on the road is driving poorly because of the rain. Monica is getting completely caught up in her stressful story—and most of it isn't even true!

If Monica were asked whether she is causing her own stress, she would probably answer, "No!" (It's the husband, kids, other drivers etc.) As is the case for most of us, this is how her mind chatters on most of the time, and she's not even aware of it. She believes her thoughts and doesn't question them. Like most of us, Monica blames her life circumstances, not her thoughts, for her stress.

So much of what causes us stress has to do with the thoughts we think, the beliefs we hold without question, our regrets about the past and our fears about the future. Most people identify completely with the thoughts in their minds. They believe they *are* their thoughts, beliefs, worries, fears and stresses about the past and the future. Tolle explains that once we are able to step back and watch those thoughts, we can see that they're just the mind and ego chattering away. When we become aware of this, we can use mindfulness practices to shift our attention to the present moment.

Some people believe that being mindful means having an empty mind, but this isn't the case for most of us, who couldn't stop our mental chatter even if our lives depended on it! For many, simply becoming aware of the chatter and tuning in to a different state of consciousness can make a profound difference in reducing stress. The goal is to develop the ability to calm the mind and body even when life gets crazy. This will translate to better health, better relationships, and better access to libido.

Jon Kabat-Zinn is another best-selling author (most notably *Coming to Our Senses* and *Wherever You Go, There You Are*) who has written extensively about mindfulness and has conducted important scientific research on how mindfulness can improve health. He points out that, "There is nothing weird or out of the ordinary about meditating or meditation. It is just about paying attention in your life as if it really mattered. And it might help to keep in mind that, while it is really nothing out of the ordinary, nothing particularly special, mindfulness is at the same time extraordinarily special and utterly transformative."

Frantically busy women may imagine that even a little bit of time practicing meditation or yoga is too much. I know—I've been in that space myself.

Let me assure you: if you take a half-hour to practice mindfulness, or even a couple of hours to go to a class to help you learn to integrate mindfulness into your life, your laundry will still be there when you finish. All that you left undone will, in all likelihood, be right where it was before. The rewards of taking that time are huge. Everything—sex, relationships, even doing the laundry—will change in a positive way as a result of mindfulness practices. As you practice mindfulness, which is primarily about directing your attention and disengaging from the mind's endless chatter, it becomes second nature and becomes integrated into all that you do.

I don't mean to advise you to simply accept your lot no matter what. I'm not suggesting that any time you find yourself overburdened, overcommitted or in a situation that is causing you a lot of stress, you should just become more mindful! If change needs to happen, make it happen. You're the best judge of that in your own life. But by learning and practicing mindfulness as you go, you'll be better able to discern what needs to change and how to take effective action to make the change.

Yes, life can be stressful and crazy. Yes, hormones can fall out of balance in midlife, which can strongly impact libido. When relationship difficulties are in the way, the idea of sex can seem roughly as enjoyable as doing yet another load of laundry. But you don't have to wait for life to calm down, for hormones to be perfectly balanced, or perfect intimacy to be achieved to start bringing your libido back. The best way back to great sex is to start *now*—wherever you are.

The keys to having an enjoyable love life at any age are time, attention and *in*tention. Make the time. Give your partner the gift of your attention. Even when things aren't going well, *hold the intention* to have the kind of sexual connection that will bring joy, health and fun.

This intention extends past the actual time spent making love. Out of that intention, mindfulness becomes a habit, schedules get made, and techniques are learned. This intention might also inspire a few visits to a sex therapist, couples therapist or workshop designed to deepen intimacy between you and your partner.

Tantra

Tantra evolved out of a set of Hindu and Buddhist spiritual beliefs and practices in the first few centuries A.D. and today is considered to be one of the many forms of yoga. The main emphasis of Tantra is that an individual, using mindfulness, visualization, breathing exercises and sometimes chanting, can purposefully channel energy within the body to achieve deeply pleasurable and even ecstatic experiences. The word *tantra* is Sanskrit for "weaving" or "loom."

Tantra is not just about sex but has become popular in the West as a means of heightening sexual experiences and improving sexual relationships. It can be done alone or with a partner. Practicing Tantra on your own can dramatically improve your sex life, even if your partner doesn't practice it with you.

A great introduction to Tantra is Barbara Carrellas' book, *Urban Tantra* (Celestial Arts, 2007) or the classic book on Tantra by Margot Anand *The Art of Sexual Ecstasy: The Path of Sacred Sexuality for Western Lovers* (Jeremy Tarcher, 1989). In many communities, experienced teachers offer Tantra classes or private instruction; videos and audio classes are also widely available.

Awakening the senses

Another kind of mindfulness is to remember, throughout the day, and during sex with yourself or your partner, to become aware of the senses: listen, look, feel, smell and taste:

- Taste - When you eat, remove distractions such as the TV and really taste your food; move it around in your mouth, chew it thoroughly, and breathe through your nose to enhance your sense of taste. (This is also a great weight loss strategy.)

- Smell - Flowers, essential oils, food, the tea you're sipping, your partner's neck, even your own scent after a workout.

- Listen - To music, birdsong, drips from a faucet, sounds of conversation, rustling leaves, your own breath.

- Feel - The sensation of fabrics, the breeze, a pet's fur against your skin, the weight of your body resting on a chair.

Mindfulness and sex

A key to remember with mindfulness is that it's a *practice*. Doing it once in a while is good, but doing it daily will do much more to shift stress levels and the ability to refocus the mind and tune into the body. As it becomes habitual, it will become part of who you are, and you will always have access to it no matter where you are or what you are doing. Stress will actually become a reminder to shift your attention to mindfulness. Once you have established your mindfulness practice, use this new level of awareness to help yourself become present in the moment, "get in the mood," and enjoy the sensual and sexual aspects of your relationship.

Whatever kind of sexual activity you and your partner choose, bring mindfulness and sensory awareness to it. Drink in the look, scent and texture of your partner's body. Attune yourself to the sensation of kissing and touching, and to how the surfaces around you feel when your body touches them. Pay attention to your own breathing and your partner's breathing. Try breathing together. When stressful thoughts intrude, shift to mindfulness.

Keep your eyes open and look at your partner at least some of the time during intimacy. While most of us automatically close our eyes during these times, keeping them open helps maintain awareness.

The rewards of bringing mindfulness to sex are many. Enjoyment is enhanced. Overall stress decreases. Intimacy between partners is strengthened. Mindfulness is a skill that can be learned and practiced by everyone.

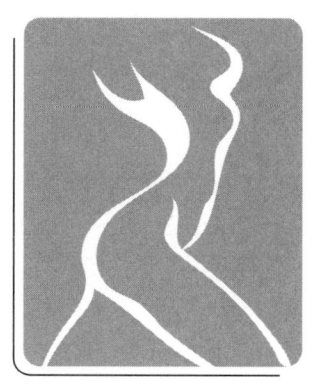

CHAPTER 9

Pro-Libido Lifestyle – Nutrition, Supplements and Exercise

Karen had just turned 50 when she first came to see me. When I wished her a happy birthday, she rolled her eyes. "Yeah, right. Happy. I'm menopausal. I can't poop. I have heartburn. My joints hurt all the time, even though I don't exercise. *At. All.*"

She was serious, but I couldn't help laughing at her delivery. "When my husband gets done complaining that I won't have sex with him, he goes to sleep and saws great big *logs* all night. Sexy! I usually just give up trying to sleep through the noise and go sit at the computer 'til 2 a.m., writing emails, reading the news, eating junk and drinking caffeine-free diet soda. Yay! It's a happy life."

When I stopped laughing, I got serious with Karen. "You might have been able to do fine with too little sleep, no exercise, and a poor diet when you were 35—maybe even when you were 40," I told her. "But those days are over."

We worked on Karen's sleep patterns first, putting her on a sleep schedule that got her eight to nine hours of sleep per night. Once she felt more rested and stopped with the late-night junk-food snacking, her heartburn improved and she felt more energetic during the day. This enabled her to start and stick with an exercise program. Exercise helped her move her bowels more efficiently, as did some dietary changes that increased the fiber and nutrient density of her meals. A nutritional supplement program came next, which improved her energy even more.

Within a few weeks, we were able to start weaning her off the antidepressants that had been suppressing her sex drive. After a few months of eating the diet I recommended, she was also able to quit taking the cholesterol-lowering drug that was contributing to her low libido. When Karen's husband got with her program, his snoring improved dramatically, and they began to enjoy taking walks and lifting weights together.

Aging can help to sink libido, but so can poor diet, late nights, prescription drugs and lack of exercise. Because we're all aging whether we like it or not, we need to focus on what we can change. Like Karen, you can make small shifts in lifestyle over time to create enormously beneficial changes.

Small Changes Add Up to Big Benefits

Hormone replacement therapy is only one part of my program to achieve the best possible state of physical health and restore libido. The rest of my program is about providing the information and motivation to make lifestyle changes, including a healthy diet and exercising at least three times a week. "I wish I could do it for you," I often say. "But I can't. It's all up to you."

Yes, as we get older, our bodies slow down a bit. Digestion can become less efficient, aches and pains may come up as joints lose suppleness. Muscle is more easily lost and fat is more easily gained. Although these changes are part of the natural progression of aging, they can be minimized through good nutrition, exercise and nutritional supplements. In youth, sex drive is strong enough to override the desire-dampening effect of unhealthy choices, but with the passing of years it takes energy and attention to keep the sexual fires burning.

Andrew Goldstein, M.D., is an expert on the science and medicine of sexuality and co-author of the book *Reclaiming Desire: 4 Keys to Finding Your Lost Libido*, (Rodale, 2004) in which he reminds us, "Your libido is incredibly sensitive; it knows when your body isn't receiving adequate nutrition, exercise, or sleep. If you're like most women, you're falling short in at least one of these core components of physical health. Your willingness and commitment to work at correcting any underlying deficiency likely will have a direct, positive impact on your sex drive."

Overcoming resistance to change

One of my first homework assignments for most of my Sex Drive Solution patients is a change in diet, and this is also where I meet the most resistance. I'm not a warm and fuzzy type when it comes to making lifestyle changes. "Just do it," is my advice.

There is little mystery surrounding the fact that so many people resist making real and lasting changes in the foods they eat. For most Americans, eating isn't just about simple sustenance; it's about celebration, reward, comfort and stress release. Food industry advertising cleverly (and largely unconsciously) reinforces the association between emotions and eating. Processed and fast foods lure us in with carefully crafted addictive tastes and textures, then deliver poor nutrition and a hefty dose of chemicals in the form of preservatives and artificial flavors and colorings. There's a learning curve to buying and preparing healthy whole foods, not to mention the challenge of convincing the rest of the family to jump on the healthy lifestyle bandwagon.

Exercise has its own set of challenges. Finding the time is hard enough, but then there's the bottom-line truth that some of us just don't like to work out. Creating a routine of daily or near-daily exercise can be an uphill struggle for those who haven't developed the habit early in life.

Jillian Michaels is transforming people's lives on reality TV with her no-nonsense approach to exercise and weight loss. In her book, *Master Your Metabolism* (Empowered Media 2009) she says, "Forget that 'walk across parking lots' and 'take the stairs' fitness advice. You can't lose weight in ten-minute bursts of exercise. No, you need to get to the gym, work your ass off when you're there, and get the job done. ...Do it even if you hate it. I do! But just like you work to pay the mortgage or your car payment, you do the work in the gym to protect your most healthy asset: a healthy body. Once you're on a steady path with exercise, you'll automatically feel less stress."

Let me say right now that once exercise is integrated into your life you'll wonder how you ever got by without it, even if it's just a walk around the block.

Keep in mind as you read on that there's an ideal level of change, which is what I'll describe here and what I recommend to my patients, but *even small changes can make a very big difference.* We're not trying to shed 10 pounds in ten days or turn you into a fitness spokesmodel. This is about changing ingrained habits gently, gradually and permanently. Consistent and strategic changes work better than sudden 180-degree shifts, because they can be maintained.

When Karen gave up drinking diet soda, her health improved. It improved even further when she managed to get on a regular sleep schedule. And every time she chose to switch out an unhealthy meal or snack for a healthier one, she felt benefits. When she got around to adding exercise, she felt even better.

When my patients muster enough motivation to go ahead and put even small pieces of the advice in this chapter into motion in their lives, they feel *so much better*. Their energy levels rise, they lose weight, their skin looks better, and their digestive systems work better. All of these changes have a positive impact on libido.

Once my patients experience the positive difference that a healthier lifestyle makes, any lapse has noticeable consequences. They go ahead and eat the way they once did on Christmas or at a wedding, and soon after they remember why they made the shift to that new dietary default. Their bodies are more sensitive to the unhealthy effects of the foods they've been avoiding. Those foods were having these effects all along, but now they can really feel the difference their nutritional choices make in their well-being.

Let's look in more detail at how the foods you eat affect your body and why certain foods are better for promoting libido than others.

The Pro-Libido Nutrition Plan: An Overview

No one way of eating works for everyone. The key is to find a way to eat that makes sense for your body, your budget and your lifestyle, while sticking to a few basic guidelines:

- Eat foods as they are found in nature whenever possible.
- Eat foods and combinations of foods that maintain blood sugar balance.

- Identify foods to which you're sensitive and eliminate them.
- Eat enough calories, but not too many.
- Eat foods that reduce inflammation.

I'll go into depth about these four elements throughout the rest of this chapter.

Eat foods the way nature makes them

The food industry has taken to adding a few isolated vitamins or a couple of grams of fiber to highly processed foods and calling them healthy or nutritious. But food manufacturers can't reproduce the combinations of nutrients found in whole foods. In order to make a processed food taste good, sugar, salt, unhealthy fats, preservatives, colorings and flavorings have to be added.

Natural, synergistic combinations of nutrients are the secret ingredients that make whole foods so good for our health. A truly healthy diet is made up of whole foods that are naturally packed full of nutrients: vitamins, minerals, phytochemicals by the hundreds, fiber and healthy fats.

The Pro Libido Nutrition Plan: Tips for Eating Foods the Way Nature Intended

- Follow author Michael Pollan's dictum about what to eat: "If your grandmother wouldn't recognize it as food, don't eat it."
- Shop the outside perimeter of the market for the healthiest choices.
- Shop at your local farmer's market whenever possible.
- Avoid prepared foods in bags, cellophane wrappers, or other fancy packaging.

- If you are considering buying a packaged food, read the label; if it has any ingredient you don't recognize as food, put it back.

- Avoid foods with artificial colorings.

- Avoid artificial sweeteners.

- Avoid foods that are preserved with nitrites or nitrates.

Preparing delicious meals with whole-food ingredients may be a learning curve for those who are used to intensely flavored processed foods that require little to no preparation. Keep in mind that the less a food is cooked, the more nutrients it retains. Keep things simple. Eat vegetables raw in salads and as snacks, or try them steamed or briefly stir-fried. Bake chicken or fish in the oven with a little olive oil and fresh herbs. Play around with spices and herbs. For great ideas try Mark Bittman's book, *How To Cook Everything: 2,000 Simple Recipes for Great Food* (Wiley, 2008).

Good carbs, bad carbs

One of the most difficult parts of the eating shift I recommend is giving up two kinds of food that have become, for most, dietary staples: foods made with white flour and foods high in sugar. We love our bagels, muffins, scones, cookies, sugary coffee drinks and sweetened yogurt! Many of the foods we believe to be healthy are loaded with sugars we don't know about until we start reading labels. But the effect these foods have on blood sugar levels is harmful in too many ways for us to keep eating them several times a day—at least if we expect to maintain libido, energy and good blood flow for decades to come.

The digestive system breaks down the food we eat into basic building blocks: fats, carbohydrates, proteins, vitamins, minerals and other nutrients. Carbohydrates break down and are absorbed into the body faster than protein or fat.

Some carbohydrates are "simpler" than others, which means they are broken down and absorbed more quickly, which leads to unstable blood sugar. Foods made from white flour or with lots of added sugar are examples of simple carbohydrates. If these simpler carbs aren't combined with other foods that contain protein and fat—both of which slow this process down—a big load of sugar is quickly dumped into the bloodstream. Complex carbs such as whole grains, vegetables, beans and fruit break down more slowly. Blood sugar rises more slowly after we eat them.

Right next to the place where the stomach opens up into the small intestine sits the pancreas. It has two jobs: it makes digestive enzymes that help digest food, and it makes a hormone called *insulin*. Insulin's job is to move sugars out of the bloodstream and into the cells of the body. When blood sugar levels rise, a healthy pancreas responds by releasing insulin, which lowers blood sugar.

When you eat simple carbs—especially when you eat them alone, without protein, fat or more complex carbs—the rise in blood sugar is steep and sudden, and the insulin response is just as steep and sudden. Blood sugar rises and then falls quickly, which can cause spaciness, shakiness, and a surge of cortisol and other stress hormones. Stressed and tired, the body sends the brain a message that it needs more refined carbs or sugar to energize it and calm it down.

Over time, this pattern leads to weight gain, lack of energy, mood swings and addiction to carbohydrate-rich foods. Over years, these fluctuations can potentially lead to a condition called *insulin resistance*, where body cells stop "listening" to the message of insulin (which is to allow sugars in the blood to pass into the cells). Blood sugars stay high despite stronger and stronger surges of insulin from the pancreas. If the same dietary pattern continues, insulin resistance will probably become type 2 diabetes, which you and your libido are better off without.

Chronically high blood sugar damages the inner walls of blood vessels. High blood sugars and high insulin levels (known as pre-diabetes) and type 2 diabetes are major risk factors for heart disease, stroke and *peripheral vascular disease*, in which blood vessels that feed the feet and legs become clogged. Men with pre-diabetes or type 2 diabetes are at much higher risk of having erectile dysfunction than men with normal blood sugars. Women with type 2 diabetes are at higher risk of sexual dysfunction than women without it. Pre-diabetes and diabetes increase inflammation throughout the body (more on this in the next section).

Pre-diabetes and diabetes are significant problems for Americans. According to the National Diabetes Information Clearinghouse (NDIC), over 25 percent of adults 20 and older are pre-diabetic. That's about 57 million adults. Of adults aged 60 and up, the NDIC found that 35.4 percent were pre-diabetic. About 21 million Americans have type 2 diabetes.

Type 2 diabetes is all about what we eat. Some who develop it find they can control it without medications just by radically changing what they eat. You're better off changing what you eat *before* developing this disease, which can prevent it entirely. *All* medications used to control type 2 diabetes have serious side effects, and *all* of them become less effective over time.

To level out blood sugar peaks and valleys, I advise patients to eat fewer carbs in general and to eat carbs that are lower on the *glycemic index* (GI). The glycemic index is a measurement of how fast a carbohydrate causes blood sugars to rise. Pure glucose (simple sugar) has a GI of 100; spinach has a GI of 15; white bread has a GI of 71, while whole-grain bread has a GI of 50. The best carbs have a GI of 50 or lower. A GI of 50 to 70 is intermediate, and the carbs to avoid run the gamut from 70 to 100.

Best Low-to-Intermediate Glycemic Index Carbohydrates

Low Glycemic Food	Glycemic Index
Artichoke	<15
Asparagus	<15
Avocado	<15
Broccoli	<15
Cauliflower	<15
Celery	<15
Cucumber	<15
Eggplant	<15
Lettuce, all varieties	<15
Green beans	<15
Peppers, all varieties	<15
Snow peas	<15
Spinach	<15
Zucchini/summer squash	<15
Tomatoes	15
Cherries	22
Plums	24
Grapefruit	25
Pearled barley	25
Agave nectar (if you need a sweetener, this is the one I recommend; or try stevia, an herbal sweetener that has no effect on blood sugar)	27
Peaches	28
Dried apricots	31
Soy milk	30
Carrots (raw)	35
Apples	36
Pears	36

Low Glycemic Food	Glycemic Index
Whole grain pasta	37
Carrots (cooked)	39
Canned chickpeas	42
Grapes	43
Oranges	43
Canned pinto beans	45
Old-fashioned (slow-cooking) oatmeal	49
Canned kidney beans	52
Kiwi	52
Orange juice, not from concentrate (from-concentrate has slightly higher GI of 57)	52
Bananas	53
Sweet potatoes	54
Brown rice	55

One easy way to determine whether a carb is good or bad is to look for color. When it comes to grains, choose those that are brown or have more color (such as whole-grain breads and yams) over white (white bread, white potatoes). Generally, the deeper the natural color, the more likely it contains carbohydrates that fall low on the glycemic index scale. Some exceptions: beets, peas and corn—all of which are pretty colorful—all have high GIs. Don't be fooled by the label "whole wheat," which generally means brown-colored white bread. Look for "whole grain" bread.

The Pro-Libido Nutrition Plan: Guidelines for Blood Sugar Balance

- Small, frequent meals are best for blood sugar balancing and help keep adrenals as healthy as possible; aim for three meals and two to three snacks per day.

- I am tough on "brown carbs" such as bread, pasta and rice. I recommend that my patients have no more than 1 serving a day. Sprouted grain breads are better than whole grains.

- Eat any other carbs in the form of low-GI vegetables (mostly) and fruits. This will provide you will all the fiber you need.

- Look for foods with lots of color and texture — crunchy fruits and vegetables are generally lower GI than soft fruits and vegetables, and they contain more nutrients.

- Any time you eat a carbohydrate-rich food, combine it with protein and fat to balance its effect on blood sugars: an apple and some walnuts, greens with olive oil vinaigrette and sliced chicken or salmon, celery with almond butter.

- If kicking sugar seems completely out of the question, know that the first few days are the hardest; after two weeks, you won't miss it anymore!

Food Sensitivities

Like Karen, whose story began this chapter, many of my patients complain of digestive symptoms when they come to see me. Bloating, indigestion, gas and constipation are some of the more common issues. The first step that I strongly suggest is to eliminate dairy and wheat from the diet for a period of four to six weeks. This can be challenging, but after a few weeks it will be cause for celebration, as the pounds drop and the energy rises.

Food sensitivities can be traced back to a reaction that happens in the intestinal tract. The lining of the small intestine is coated with immune cells that are responsible for identifying and eliminating unwanted substances in the foods we eat. It's estimated that 70 percent of the immune system is in the gut. Many people's intestinal immune systems react to proteins found in wheat and dairy, which are staple foods for Americans from an early age. The proteins in wheat are called *gluten*, and many other grains also contain this gluey substance. Over time this immune reaction will cause irritation and inflammation in the gut, which creates tiny holes in the wall of the small intestine. This situation—known as "leaky gut"—then allows undigested food particles to pass into the bloodstream. The immune system throughout the body is triggered by the presence of these seemingly foreign substances, causing body-wide inflammation and a long list of symptoms, including chronic fatigue, headaches, joint pain, brain fog and recurrent sinus problems. Even when this sensitivity doesn't cause outright symptoms, it does drain energy and create chronic irritation in the digestive tract. You're much more likely to feel sexy if you're not bloated, gassy and unhappy!

A food sensitivity is not the same as a food allergy. An allergic reaction to a food is immediate (hives, sneezing, itchy throat, watery eyes). Sensitivities are delayed reactions that make causes difficult to trace. Because wheat and dairy sensitivities are so common (some estimates find that 80 percent of adults have some level of sensitivity to one or both of these foods), the most sensible approach is to try eliminating them for a while to see if any symptoms or problems clear up as a result.

A person who has a positive thyroid antibody test is more likely to be gluten-sensitive than someone with normal thyroid function. When the immune system starts to attack the thyroid gland it may be doing so in part because of immune sensitivity to gluten. Eliminating gluten can help normalize thyroid function for some people.

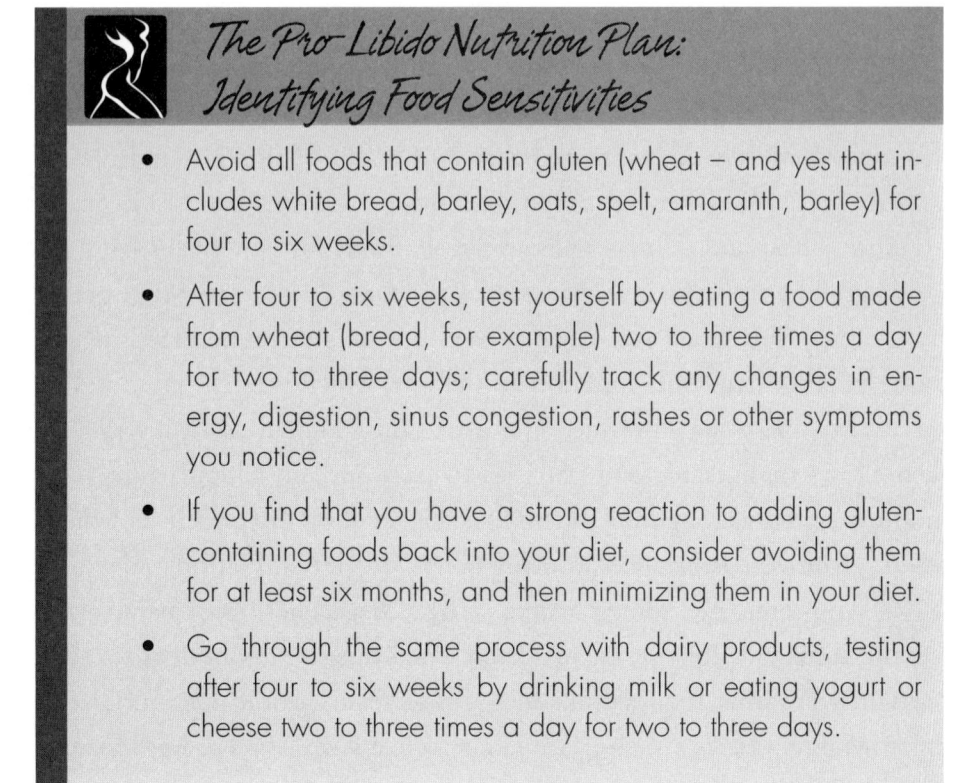

The Pro-Libido Nutrition Plan: Identifying Food Sensitivities

- Avoid all foods that contain gluten (wheat — and yes that includes white bread, barley, oats, spelt, amaranth, barley) for four to six weeks.

- After four to six weeks, test yourself by eating a food made from wheat (bread, for example) two to three times a day for two to three days; carefully track any changes in energy, digestion, sinus congestion, rashes or other symptoms you notice.

- If you find that you have a strong reaction to adding gluten-containing foods back into your diet, consider avoiding them for at least six months, and then minimizing them in your diet.

- Go through the same process with dairy products, testing after four to six weeks by drinking milk or eating yogurt or cheese two to three times a day for two to three days.

In my practice, women often wonder what they *can* eat if they're avoiding these dietary staples. Your local health food store is a good place to find a variety of crackers and breads without gluten. Non-gluten-containing grains include rice, quinoa and millet. Corn doesn't contain gluten but is high on the glycemic index and is also high on the list of foods that can cause inflammation. Try non-gluten breads and pastas made from rice and dairy substitutes such as soy, rice and almond milks and cheeses, but be wary of overdoing it with highly processed non-gluten, non-dairy foods. They're likely to contain lots of sugar or artificial flavorings. Just because it's gluten-free and dairy-free doesn't mean it's healthy. Soy can cause indigestion in many people—I don't recommend making soy a staple of the diet. Any vegetable, fruit, nut or seed is fine; so are healthy protein sources such as eggs, fish, chicken and lean meat in moderation. Many people who can't tolerate regular wheat products find that they do fine with foods made from sprouted grains (again, try your local health food store).

Most of my patients who go through with this period of elimination and reintroduction of gluten and dairy find that they do, in fact, have sensitivities to these foods. They feel a huge difference in their energy and well-being while off of those foods, and when they go back on, old symptoms return and energy levels drop. Ultimately, I prefer that most of my patients be wheat-free and dairy-free for the long term. This doesn't mean never having these foods again, but it does mean understanding that they don't agree with your body if you make them a regular part of your diet. We all have lapses, but once it's clear that a sensitivity is there, you'll have a much better idea of what you're getting into when you fall off the wagon.

Sometimes, just quitting wheat without quitting all gluten-containing grains is enough to drastically reduce symptoms. Many people eat wheat at every meal and snack; once wheat is eliminated, it's tough to eat enough of the other gluten-containing grains (like barley and oats) to match that constant influx of a single food. Just quitting wheat may be enough to make inflammation and irritation subside despite continued eating of other grains that contain gluten. I completely understand when patients tell me how difficult it is to eliminate wheat from the diet—it seems to be in everything, from soups to cereals and almost all baked goods. However, once you learn how to avoid wheat, and how to eat carbs without it, the rewards will be well worth the self-discipline it takes to take a pass on that muffin or cookie.

Putting Fats in Perspective

Despite all the bad press it's gotten in the past few decades, fat is an important part of a healthy diet. When fat was condemned as a threat to health, food manufacturers processed the daylights out of natural foods to remove it, at which point they advertised them as healthier choices.

Nutritional research has clearly shown that a low-fat diet is *not* good for health. Although the processed trans-fats (e.g. hydrogenated oils) and non-food-derived fats like cottonseed oil should be avoided, there really are no "bad" fat foods. Any fat is unhealthy when eaten in excess. Americans tend to over-eat the saturated fats found in meat, and the vegetable oils found in processed foods. That means most of us need to eat more of the fats found in fish, nuts and seeds, olive oil and avocadoes. Cold pressed extra virgin olive oil seems to be a particularly safe and healthy oil.

It is also not true that eating fat will make you fat. Some fats, such as coconut oil, can promote weight loss. Eating *excess* fat will make you fat, but eating excess carbs and sugar will also make you fat.

And while we're on the subject of fat myths, it is not true that eating cholesterol-containing foods will raise your cholesterol levels. Your liver makes 75 percent of your cholesterol and the rest comes from food. Any excess cholesterol is easily disposed of by the body *unless you eat it in excess!* Yes, if you look at your blood an hour after eating a greasy burger and fries, you will see a lot of fat in the blood, but in a healthy body that is gone within a few hours. I'm not advocating that you eat a greasy burger and fries, I'm just putting fat and cholesterol in perspective. Furthermore, it is not saturated fat per se that clogs your arteries, it is the inflammation caused by eating *excess* red meat, excess vegetable oils, and excess carbs and sugar. The take-home message here is all about excess.

Fat and inflammation

When we are injured or come down with the flu, the immune system creates an inflammatory response to heal the wound or to fight off the bug that is causing the infection. The swelling and redness of a sprained ankle and the fever that spikes during the flu are both examples of the kind of inflammation that heals. But in a body that's fed too much fat and simple carbohydrate, the balance of the inflammatory process is tipped. At the cellular level, excess fats and simple carbs are transformed into chemicals that create a chronic state of low-grade inflammation.

Low-grade inflammation is associated with a higher risk of heart attack, stroke, type 2 diabetes, kidney disease and some cancers. In Alzheimer's disease, inflammation gradually eats away at the hardware of memory much like a smoldering fire eats away at firewood.

Obesity makes this inflammatory imbalance worse, which helps to explain why it's believed to shorten lifespan and raise the risk of age-related diseases. As recently as the 1990s, it was believed that fat cells were just inactive repositories for extra calories. Now it's known that when fat cells become overstuffed, they react by producing chemical messengers called *cytokines*, which increase inflammation throughout the body. A person who is obese is in a constantly elevated state of inflammation, and this is taxing. Obesity depletes energy and by association is also likely to deplete libido.

The pro-libido eating plan is anti-inflammatory. Most everyone needs a nutrition plan that reduces inflammation. Reducing or cutting out processed foods made mostly of flour, sugar, vegetable oils and chemicals will dramatically reduce inflammation.

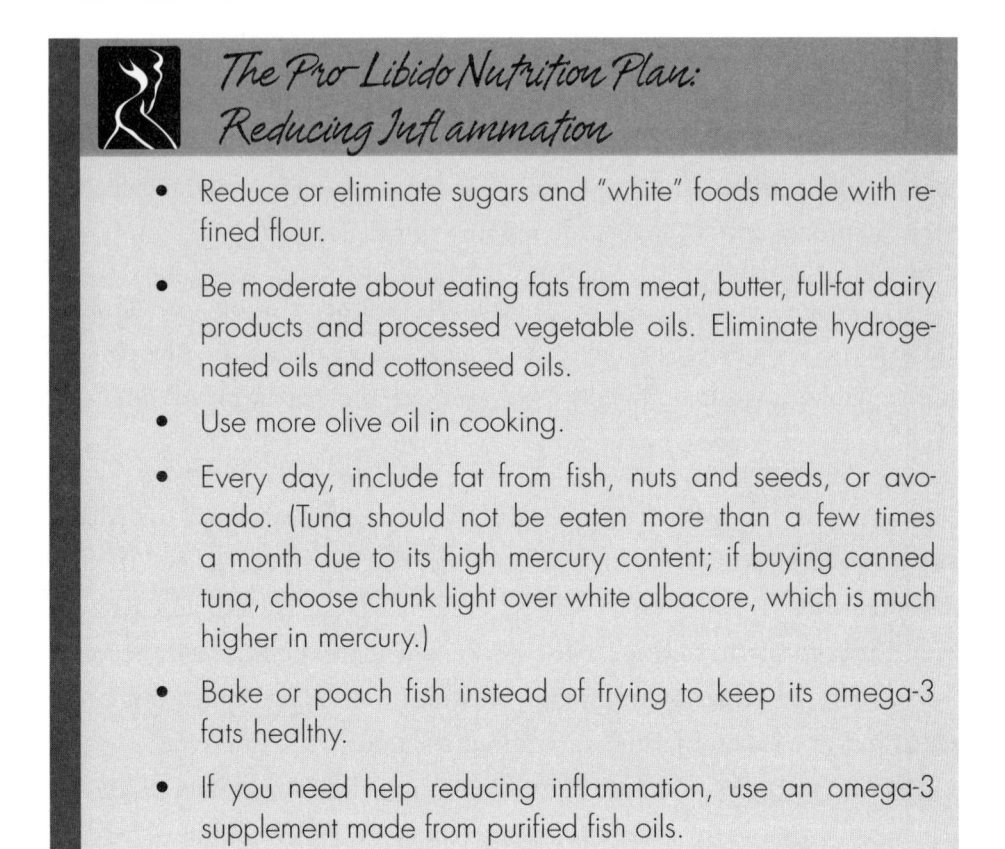

The Pro-Libido Nutrition Plan: Reducing Inflammation

- Reduce or eliminate sugars and "white" foods made with refined flour.

- Be moderate about eating fats from meat, butter, full-fat dairy products and processed vegetable oils. Eliminate hydrogenated oils and cottonseed oils.

- Use more olive oil in cooking.

- Every day, include fat from fish, nuts and seeds, or avocado. (Tuna should not be eaten more than a few times a month due to its high mercury content; if buying canned tuna, choose chunk light over white albacore, which is much higher in mercury.)

- Bake or poach fish instead of frying to keep its omega-3 fats healthy.

- If you need help reducing inflammation, use an omega-3 supplement made from purified fish oils.

Keeping Portion Sizes In Proportion

Americans' portion sizes and calorie intakes have increased dramatically in the past 40 years. Between 1971 and 2000, women's daily intake of calories rose from 1,542 a day to 1,877, and the average woman is burning fewer calories today than a woman of the 1970s. Men's portion sizes have increased even more than this, with no corresponding increase in physical activity. It's no wonder that 66 percent of Americans are overweight and 30 percent of them obese. The rate of obesity has doubled since the 1980s—a decade when, according to the Centers for Disease Control and Prevention, the average adult gained eight pounds!

Weight loss is a common goal for women who come to see me for hormone balancing. I support patients in this when they are actually overweight or obese because carrying too many extra pounds fatigues the body, saps libido, and sets us up for illness and faster aging. When nutrient-dense whole foods replace low-nutrient, processed, high-carbohydrate foods, and when foods are combined in the way I recommend, weight loss tends to happen on its own as the body moves into a more balanced state.

Research on weight gain throughout the female lifespan shows that a menopausal woman is better off with a few extra pounds—that being a little "overweight" may actually be good for health in menopause. This is probably because estrogen is made in fat cells. Ever notice how a man with a lot of belly fat starts to look a little feminine? It's because those extra pounds around the midsection are estrogen factories.

For a premenopausal woman, excess weight can cause estrogen dominance (see Chapter 4 for details), and for these women, weight loss can help improve health and libido. But women who are thin *after* menopause are more likely to have problems related to estrogen deficiency, including osteoporosis and vaginal dryness. A little extra fat is actually good for libido in a menopausal woman. While being too fat or too thin is inarguably unhealthy, there's a huge individual variation in what constitutes healthy weight. A healthy weight shouldn't be solely determined by a scale or a chart, it should be based on factors such as energy and activity levels. If you're active, eating wholesome foods in moderation and have balanced hormones, chances are your weight is just fine, even if you don't have the body of a celebrity.

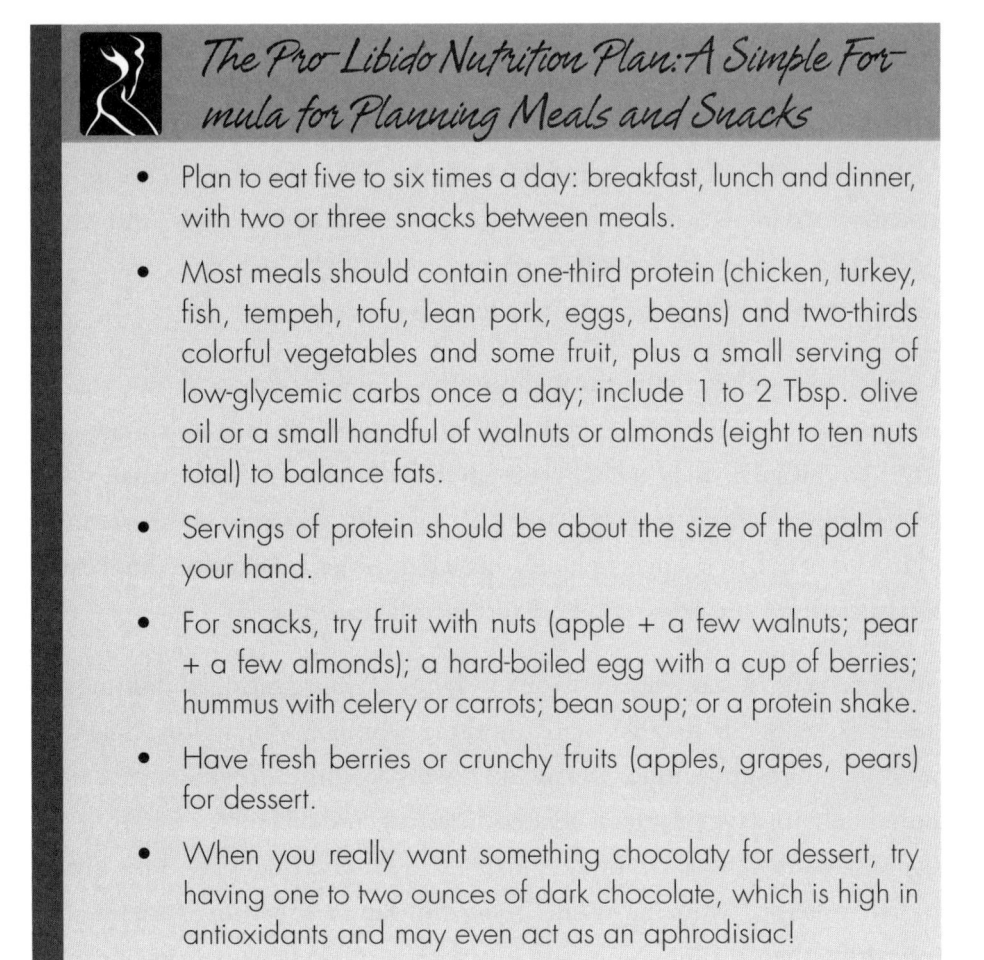

The Pro-Libido Nutrition Plan: A Simple Formula for Planning Meals and Snacks

- Plan to eat five to six times a day: breakfast, lunch and dinner, with two or three snacks between meals.

- Most meals should contain one-third protein (chicken, turkey, fish, tempeh, tofu, lean pork, eggs, beans) and two-thirds colorful vegetables and some fruit, plus a small serving of low-glycemic carbs once a day; include 1 to 2 Tbsp. olive oil or a small handful of walnuts or almonds (eight to ten nuts total) to balance fats.

- Servings of protein should be about the size of the palm of your hand.

- For snacks, try fruit with nuts (apple + a few walnuts; pear + a few almonds); a hard-boiled egg with a cup of berries; hummus with celery or carrots; bean soup; or a protein shake.

- Have fresh berries or crunchy fruits (apples, grapes, pears) for dessert.

- When you really want something chocolaty for dessert, try having one to two ounces of dark chocolate, which is high in antioxidants and may even act as an aphrodisiac!

More Pro-Libido Nutrition Guidelines

Drink plenty of water; six to eight glasses a day is best for most people. Just getting enough fluid into your body can plump skin and improve energy levels. Avoid or limit caffeine, which stresses the adrenals. Avoid sodas—even diet sodas, which don't aid in weight loss; some studies actually find that diet sodas encourage weight *gain*. I can't even count the number of women I have seen who have lost weight just by giving up soda, including diet soda. Both sodas and caffeine are dehydrating. Avoid preservatives (especially nitrates and nitrites) and foods and beverages colored with dyes.

Make healthy eating a family affair; at the very least, team up with your partner to plan good eating together. It's tough to be the only one eating well while everyone else keeps bringing home bags of fast food. You might find a healthy nutrition/workout buddy among your girlfriends. Collect and exchange recipes and ideas to keep healthy eating fun. Have a potluck where you and your friends can share your latest healthy culinary masterpieces.

Bring mindfulness to your meals. Instead of wolfing food down, eat slowly and pay attention to what you're eating. Break the habit of eating while driving, watching TV, surfing the Web or reading. Take small bites and chew slowly. Whenever possible, eat without distractions. At meditation retreats, meals are often eaten in silence to help participants be more aware of what they're eating. I'm not suggesting that you insist on silence when you sit down with your family or partner to eat, but it's definitely okay to let a little quiet settle in while you savor your food! Try to avoid stressful topics of conversation at the family dinner table.

The appeal of processed, heavy or otherwise unhealthy food falls away when you eat mindfully. And if you do decide to eat French fries or cookies, eating them mindfully will get you to a place of satisfaction before you gobble down too many.

Drinking alcohol is okay on the pro-libido nutrition plan. Limit yourself to five to seven drinks a week; red wine seems to have the most evidence in terms of benefits to health. Drinking three or more of those drinks at a sitting is considered binge drinking in a woman, and that's harmful to your health (obviously). Have no more than two alcoholic drinks in one day.

Pro-libido nutritional supplements

By shifting to the foods recommended in this chapter, you'll get a boost in your intake of the vitamins, minerals, balanced fats and other nutrients you need. Adding a few nutritional supplements helps cover all your bases.

Start with a multivitamin. The average one-a-day multivitamin supplement contains the Recommended Daily Allowance (RDA) of a handful of nutrients, which most people think is all that's necessary for good health and disease prevention. But getting the RDA actually means getting just enough of a nutrient to prevent vitamin deficiency diseases like scurvy, rickets or beriberi. In most Westernized countries, these kinds of outright deficiency diseases are very, very rare. A big gap exists between bare-minimum nutrient requirements (the RDA) and the amount known to help prevent disease, slow the aging process, and promote energy and health.

Don't worry about getting too much of any of these nutrients from your multi. Any nutrient supplied at 200 or more percent of the RDA has been proven safe at that dose.

The box below outlines some specifications to help you choose a higher-potency multivitamin. You'll see that doses of some important nutrients, including the minerals calcium and magnesium, are well below or right at the RDA. This is either because most experts recommend supplementing these nutrients separately because there's more than enough in the average diet or because no health benefit of higher doses has been found. I recommend specific forms of nutrients when research suggests that a particular form is better absorbed or utilized by the body. Many high-quality multivitamins will include ingredients not in this table, but these are the most important.

Daily Multivitamin/Mineral for the Pro-Libido Nutrition Plan

Name and Form of Nutrient	Daily Recommended Dose	% DV/RDA
Vitamin A as natural mixed carotenoids and palmitate	15,000 IU (International Units)	300
Vitamin C as ascorbic acid	1,000 mg	1667
Vitamin D3 as cholecalciferol	1,000 IU	250
Vitamin E as d-alpha tocopherol succinate	200 IU	667
Vitamin E as mixed tocopherols	100 IU	*
Vitamin K as phytonadione	100 mcg (micrograms)	125
Thiamine (vitamin B1)	50 mg	3,333
Riboflavin (vitamin B2)	50 mg	2,941
Niacin	50 mg	250
Pyridoxine (vitamin B6)	75 mg	3,750
Folic Acid	800 mcg	200
Vitamin B12 as methylcobalamin	1,000 mcg	1,667
Biotin	400 mcg	133
Pantothenic Acid as d-calcium pantothenate	300 mg	3,000
Calcium as di-calcium malate	200 mg	20
Magnesium as d-magnesium malate, ascorbate or glycinate, or a mixture	400 mg	100
Zinc as glycinate or chelate	20	133
Selenium	200 mcg	266
Copper as glycinate or chelate	2 mg	100
Manganese	5 mg	250
Chromium	400 mcg	333
Molybdenum	50 mcg	67
Potassium as citrate	100 mg	3

There's no way to get all of these nutrients in ideal doses in a one-a-day supplement. Expect to swallow three to six multivitamins a day to get these generous doses of nutrients into your body. Try to take vitamins with food. If vitamins upset your stomach, try those made from food concentrates. If that doesn't work, don't take them! Focus instead on eating a balanced and healthy diet of whole foods.

Omega-3 fish oils

To calm inflammation, take an omega-3 supplement every day. Fish oil is the best source of EPA and DHA—*long-chain omega-3 fatty acids*, which are the kind the body uses best to combat inflammation. Choose a fish oil made from salmon or small, cold-water ocean fish like sardines or anchovies. (Generally, the lower on the food chain the fish is, the less mercury and other toxins it picks up during its lifespan; the colder the water it lives in, the higher the fish's omega-3 fat content will be.) Check to make sure the oil has gone through a process called molecular distillation to ensure that it's been purified (this should be stated on the product's label). Also look for the term pharmaceutical grade for better quality fish oils. While there are many good brands out there, two that I recommend are Carlson's or Nordic Naturals.

Aim for 1,500 to 3,000 mg per day of EPA and DHA combined; this will probably require four to six capsules a day. Cheaper brands of fish oil contain only about 30 percent EPA and DHA, while higher-quality brands have higher content of these healthy oils. Choose a brand that contains 50 percent or more EPA and DHA. For a fish oil that contains 500 mg of fatty acids per capsule and that is 50 percent EPA/DHA, you'd need to take three to six capsules to get your daily 1,500 to 3,000 mg of omega-3. Don't take more than 3,000 mg per day without a doctor's guidance, as this can thin the blood enough to raise risk of abnormal bleeding.

Keep fish oil capsules in the refrigerator. If you find that the oil causes "fish burps" or heartburn, try freezing the capsules or buy an enteric-coated brand. Enteric-coated capsules don't break down until they get through the stomach into the small intestines, at which point they're too far along to repeat on you.

Here's what is known about the potential health benefits of long-chain omega-3 fats, based on hundreds of research studies. Adequate long-chain omega-3s:

- Reduce inflammation.

- Decrease risk of heart disease and stroke by lowering triglycerides, raising "good" HDL cholesterol levels, lowering blood pressure and decreasing formation of plaques in arteries that feed the heart and brain.

- Decrease risk of life-threatening heartbeat irregularities in people who have already had a heart attack.

- Appear to reduce risk of colon, prostate and breast cancers.

- May reduce joint stiffness and pain caused by arthritis.

- Can reduce pain from menstrual periods.

- May help maintain bone density and prevent osteoporosis.

- May positively impact mood, mental clarity, memory and attention.

If you take blood-thinning drugs or medications to lower blood sugar, adding fish oil supplements to your nutrition plan may affect the action of those medications. Let your doctor or pharmacist know you plan to add fish oil so that you can have dosages adjusted as needed. Taking omega-3s with cyclosporine (a drug given to suppress the immune system in organ transplant patients), cholesterol-lowering medicines, the acne drug Retin-

A or steroid creams for psoriasis has been found to help those medicines work better.

Vitamin D: Sunshine and supplements

Vitamin D plays a role in virtually every aspect of health. It's involved in the function of the immune system; in bone growth and maintenance; and in the regulation of cell growth and death. Lack of vitamin D causes bones to soften and is a cause of osteoporosis, osteopenia (softening bones, not quite osteoporosis), and muscle and joint pain. Over the past few years, a link between low vitamin D and increased risk of heart disease has been confirmed. Higher risk of cancer and infection has also been linked back to low vitamin D levels. Cognition and mood may also be impacted by low vitamin D. New data shows that vitamin D helps regulate blood sugar levels and may help with weight loss. And higher levels of vitamin D are associated with a lower risk of dementia.

This vitamin isn't even really a vitamin, it's a steroid hormone. When sunshine strikes the skin, vitamin D is produced in amounts far greater than that found in any food. In latitudes below the northernmost parts of the U.S., 15 minutes of sun exposure a day is enough to create as much vitamin D as a Caucasian person's body needs. A person with darker skin requires a little more sun exposure. Food sources of vitamin D are rare. Dairy products are vitamin D fortified, but we can't count on them to provide adequate levels.

A study published in 2009 found a deficiency of vitamin D in over 75 percent of the U.S. population. Over 22,000 people had their blood levels of vitamin D measured for this study. Deficiency was even more common in Asian, black and Hispanic people: about 90 percent had levels below those known to promote good health. Less time spent outdoors and obesity—which reduces vitamin D production—are the likely causes of this widespread vitamin D deficiency. The link between obesity and poor health could be due, in part, to this decreased vitamin D production. As we age, our bodies become less able to make the vitamin D we need.

Ideally, it's best to get out in the sunshine at least twice a week for 15 to 20 minutes. For those who live in latitudes above the line that can be drawn across the U.S. from northern California to Boston, this may not do the trick, as the ultraviolet rays in those areas are not strong enough for much of the year to produce adequate vitamin D. Cloud cover, shade, glass windows and sunscreen all block enough UV rays to strongly reduce vitamin D production in the skin.

I advise everyone to supplement with at least 1,000 IU per day of this vitamin in the form of vitamin D3. (Some supplements contain vitamin D2, which is not nearly as well absorbed and used by the body.) There are no risks in supplementing with this amount of vitamin D. The body makes 10,000 to 15,000 IU during a 15 to 20 minute period in the sun, sunscreen-free. The bare minimum I recommend is 1,000 IU per day.

Have a vitamin D blood test performed to see what your levels are. After supplementing for a while, get a re-test to ensure that you're getting enough of this important nutrient. It's important to measure levels of this nutrient because there is also a risk of vitamin D toxicity with higher levels of vitamin D.

Calcium and magnesium

Vitamin D promotes strong bones by helping the body to absorb more calcium from the foods we eat. It also reduces the amount of calcium lost from the body through urine. Magnesium is a mineral, like calcium, that helps to balance out and improve calcium's effects on bone health. Both calcium and magnesium play roles in the functioning of the cardiovascular system.

Supplement calcium in the form of calcium citrate or calcium hydroxyapatite. The most common form of calcium sold as a supplement is calcium carbonate, which isn't well absorbed. Supplementing with calcium carbonate over a long period of time poses a risk of kidney stones. Calcium hydroxyapatite is best at increasing bone density.

Take between 700 and 1,200 mg of calcium a day. Balance your calcium intake with 400 mg per day of magnesium, taken at bedtime. Remember to take into account the amount of calcium in the foods you eat. For example, a serving of greens may have as much as 300 mg of calcium. I recommend to my patients to supplement calcium at night and determine the amount depending on what they have gotten during the day. Many Americans are magnesium deficient and magnesium replacement has helped many of my patients with many symptoms including leg cramps and constipation. Magnesium oxide can act as a laxative; if you don't need help moving your bowels, choose a different form of magnesium. One of the forms I most recommend is the gylcinate form of magnesium. I also recommend that magnesium be taken at night because it does have a nice relaxing effect.

Other supplements I recommend

Here are a few other supplemental nutrients to round out your pro-libido nutrition plan:

Probiotics help create the best possible balance of "good bugs" in the digestive tract, which in turn will reduce unpleasant digestive symptoms like constipation, bloating and indigestion. Probiotics improve your body's ability to break down food and utilize the nutrients it contains. Supplement daily with a live probiotic that supplies 20 billion colony forming units (CFUs). Look for a supplement that contains a mix of lactobacilli, bifidobacterium and saccharomyces. Make this a daily ritual because these good bugs don't replenish themselves. Avoid highly sweetened yogurts that advertise themselves as good probiotic sources; it's easy to get the probiotics without all that sugar and dairy.

Chromium picolinate. This mineral helps keep blood sugars balanced. If you are kicking a sugar habit or know you tend to have big blood sugar rises and dips, take 600 micrograms (mcg) per day of chromium picolinate along with a half-milligram (500 mcg) of vanadyl sulfate, another mineral with blood sugar-lowering effects. These nutrients may be found in adequate amounts in a good multivitamin.

Antioxidants: resveratrol and alpha lipoic acid. Antioxidants are one of our front-line defenses against age-related diseases and premature aging. They also help mend the destructive effect of excess inflammation. In addition to the antioxidants in your multivitamin (vitamins A, C and E), take resveratrol, which is a powerful antioxidant derived from grape seeds, at a dose of 100 to 300 mg per day, and alpha-lipoic acid, which helps other antioxidants to work better and does a lot to protect the body against oxidative damage, at a dose of 300 mg per day.

For weight loss: L-carnitine and conjugated linoleic acid (CLA). Those who wish to lose weight can try taking 2,000 mg per day of L-carnitine, a fat-burning amino acid, and three grams per day of CLA, a type of fat molecule that has been found to help promote weight loss.

The Pro-Libido Workout Plan

Regular exercise absolutely improves libido. It does so by enhancing energy, improving body image, and getting blood flowing to every part of the body.

The most important—and most difficult—advice I have on the topic of exercise is this: Staying fit and energetic through midlife and beyond requires some form of cardiovascular exercise, done for at least 30 minutes *at least* three times a week. Strength training should be done just as often.

That's an hour of exercise three times a week or a half-hour six days a week. You need to commit yourself to doing something physical every day.

That's right. *Every day.*

When you do something every day, it becomes a habit. It gets easier because it's like brushing your teeth or making your bed. It's just something you do. Eventually, it gets to where you miss it when you absolutely have to skip a day. Your body starts to crave that hit of physical activity, sweat and endorphins (those "feel-good" chemicals made in the body in response to exercise).

Exercise is an essential part of maintaining quality of life. Make it part of your routine, and don't let it be disturbed unless there's an emergency—and even then, reschedule any missed workout sessions. Treat workouts like you'd treat a business meeting with an important client. No excuses!

Exercising with a buddy or in a group can really help when motivation sags. So can working with a personal trainer or DVDs of different workout programs. From my own experience, I know that the help of a personal trainer can be truly transformative. My shoulders used to slump forward, and I thought that was just how my body was put together. But when I worked with a great trainer, he showed me that my slumpy shoulders were more about muscular imbalance between back and chest muscles rather than heredity, and now my shoulders look and feel completely different. Have a trainer come to your home or gym to work with both you and your mate to help you keep your workout programs fresh and challenging.

Cardiovascular exercise burns calories and improves heart health, blood flow and muscular endurance. Walking, swimming, running, stair-climbing, jumping rope, dancing, or cycling are all types of cardio. Even doing a circuit of different strength-training exercises without resting in between can get your heart rate up high enough to qualify as cardio. (Sex can be cardiovascularly challenging, too—but we'll consider those workouts extra.)

To find out whether your chosen cardio is intense enough, get a heart rate monitor or learn to check your heart rate. Then, subtract your age from 220 to find the maximum heart (MHR) rate for a woman your age. If your heart rate is between 65 and 80 percent of that MHR, you're in your cardio zone. Keep yourself there for 30 minutes three times a week. The better conditioned you become, the more intensely you'll need to exercise to reach your target zone—and that means that your heart and lungs are getting more and more efficient.

Strength training preserves and builds bone mass and muscle. After 40, muscle won't stick around if we don't do something to convince it that it's needed! Any kind of resistance training will work: try simple pushups, sit ups and other calisthenics, weight training with dumbbells or on machines, Pilates or one of the more strenuous forms of yoga. A lot of my patients love strength bands because they are easy to do anywhere and great for travel.

Whichever mode of resistance training you choose, work each body part (arms/shoulders, chest, back, abs and legs/butt are each considered separate body parts in the world of resistance training) two times a week and work it until it's thoroughly fatigued. For example, when doing bicep curls with 5-pound dumbbells, lift the weights enough times to feel real tiredness in the arms. Then, rest and do another set. A little soreness the next day tells you that you're building muscle.

Mix things up and keep them interesting. Exercise doesn't have to be boring! It could be as simple as taking a walk and doing some pushups, situps and squats. Or you could go to a Pilates class, a yoga class, or an aerobic dance class. Try something new; train for an athletic event or sign up for ballroom dance classes with your partner. Having a goal definitely makes exercising more exciting. I recently finished my first half marathon and it was an awesome event. I had never run more than 3 to 4 miles, and within three months of training with some super terrific women to help get me through it, I managed to go the whole 13.1 miles with a smile on my face. Now I'm training for a sprint triathlon. Racing is a great way to get motivated. Consider starting with a local 5K and raising money for a great cause in conjunction with the race. The race and the fundraising may act as added encouragement to keep going on the mornings when you don't really feel like getting up to train. Just because you've never done it before doesn't mean you can't. Last year I never would have thought I could run 13 miles but I just did it, and you can do it too. I'm not much of a swimmer or biker yet but I think the courage to try is the important thing and to just get out there and "do it" as the Nike slogan says!

Women who have never exercised before get really scared at this idea of working out daily. I tell them to start out with five minutes a day or just one or two short workouts a week. Once that feels doable, I have them push it up to ten minutes, and so on.

If this reminds you of yourself, remember that whatever it takes to gradually work into a regular program is what's best for you. Forcing yourself into a sudden workout frenzy might have benefits at first, but you won't be able to keep it up. Start out slow, steady and gentle but aim for that goal of exercise every day. *Every day.*

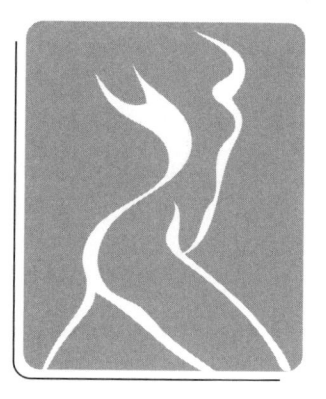

CHAPTER 10

How to Revive the Bored Libido

When Gail first came to see me, she said that her libido had been fine all the way through her 40s, and that she and her husband had enjoyed a relatively good sex life. "It wasn't exotic," she explained. "We had sex every week or so, and it was plain vanilla, but it was *good* vanilla." As Gail moved into menopause, her desire for sex evaporated. She still said yes to her husband's advances, but it didn't feel like it once did, and at times it was painful and then she felt resentful.

We did hormone testing and based on the results, I prescribed progesterone, estrogen and testosterone. When Gail returned in three months, she said that her vaginal dryness had improved, but she still just couldn't seem to get enthusiastic about having sex. After establishing that her relationship with her husband was OK, I asked Gail, "What would happen if I asked you to watch your favorite movie twice a week over and over and over again, for a year?"

"I'm sure I'd be sick of it after a few weeks," she replied.

"Yet that's what you're doing with your sex life—you've been doing the same thing with the same guy in the same bed over and over and over—maybe you're just bored!"

We talked about how Gail could bring some novelty into her sex life by creating more mindfulness, and by using some of the sex toys and techniques described in this chapter.

At first, Gail was taken aback by the idea of using sex toys, erotica, pornography, masturbation or Tantric techniques to increase her sensation and pleasure in lovemaking. She didn't see herself as the kind of woman who would buy and use a vibrator, read an erotic story, or masturbate while watching a movie that showed explicit sex. When I suggested that she and her husband create a schedule for sex and stick to it, she thought that my approach lacked romance—which she and her husband had always found to be an important aspect of their sex life together. But I made the point that if what she'd been doing until now wasn't working, these "out of the box" approaches might have a better chance of rekindling their love life.

"Okay, you're the doctor, so I guess you must know what you're talking about," she said reluctantly, "but I can't imagine going into one of those… *novelty stores*…and shopping for sex toys or dirty movies!" I reassured her that she could do her shopping online and that her purchases would arrive in discreet packaging.

The next time I saw Gail in my office, she was grinning like the Cheshire Cat. "We found some new ideas that really, *really* worked," she told me. "Thank you for being straight with me. I'd never have done any of these things unless my doctor had told me to!"

In this chapter, I'll share some practical tips for couples who are ready to hit the "refresh" button on their sex life. I'll explain why, when libidos are low, it's best to schedule sex; which toys and exercises work best to build sexual desire and sensation; and how erotica, fantasy and pornography can support a healthy sex life as long as they're used to deepen the connection between partners.

Scheduling Sex

One of the biggest hurdles I have to overcome with my Sex Drive Solution patients is acceptance of my homework assignment to schedule sex. Why is this concept so difficult for so many? Dr. Esther Perel, author of the book *Mating In Captivity: Unlocking Erotic Intelligence*, (Harper 2006) maintains that it's a form of prudishness. She explains, "The idea that sex must be spontaneous keeps us one step removed from having to will sex, to own our desire, and to express it with intent. As long as sex is something that just happens, you don't have to claim it. It's ironic that in such a willful society, willfully conjuring up sex seems obvious and crass. It embarrasses us, as if we've been caught doing something inappropriate."

Sex should be spontaneous, right? A rush of desire followed by a scramble for the bedroom, the tearing off of clothes, and then a mad melting together into a passionate embrace? And before this happens, shouldn't there be some sort of electrifying sexual tension that builds almost to the breaking point?

Sure, it should be this way—for characters in movies, steamy novels and TV shows, but in the nonfiction world of long-term relationships and aging bodies, waiting for that spontaneous moment may result in a nonexistent sex life. You might think that scheduling sex would bring on boredom, but once partners are together during their scheduled time for physical intimacy, all kinds of spontaneity and creativity can occur!

How often? This depends entirely on the couple. I've had couples who started off with scheduling sex two to three times a week, and those who felt they were making great progress by scheduling it once a month. Couples with different ideas of "how often" need to negotiate a schedule that works for both. If you and your partner can't agree on a schedule, bring in a neutral third party—preferably a counselor or a sex therapist—to help.

How about time of day? As men grow older, they may find that their erections are stronger and harder in the morning than they are at night. A man in this situation might wake up Sunday morning with a hard erection but might not be able to get hard enough for sex on Saturday night. What if the female partner prefers Saturday night after an evening out together? There's always Viagra, but in some men, the medication works better in the morning than at night. This is likely because it's usually taken after a meal at night and on an empty stomach in the morning. Levitra, another ED medication, can work better in this circumstance.

Three hours is usually a reasonable amount of time to spend together on a sex date. No matter what transpires, stay together and engage with each other in some way for at least the allotted amount of time. If you run over, well, worse things have happened!

Once you and your partner have agreed upon a schedule, put it in your calendars. Make that time sacrosanct. Unless a serious issue comes up, *be there*.

What if you don't have a partner but are looking to revive your libido to help you find the right mate? Set up date nights anyhow, and have your dates with yourself. You can use the techniques described later in this chapter to give yourself pleasure and to prepare for the partner you're seeking.

The power of anticipation and resolving radically different libidos

One of the best aspects of planning sex is the element of anticipation. Try sending text messages ("I can't wait for our date tonight!" or something more suggestive) or planning the evening so that it can include an elegant meal and a bubble bath. Scheduled time for lovemaking helps women to clear the decks of other concerns and to bring their focus to romance. Sex on a schedule helps men who take drugs for erectile dysfunction (ED) to plan the use of their medication.

I often recommend that my patients make a list of all the things that are on their mind, including all the thoughts that might prevent them from being there in the moment during a sex date, and to physically leave the list in another room so they can create mental and physical separation from their mundane tasks.

A sex schedule that works for both partners can help resolve the issues that arise when one partner wants more sex than the other: the higher-libido partner asks and is rejected again and again and may just give up; the lower-libido partner finds herself repeatedly rejecting and feeling guilty—or begrudgingly having sex she doesn't want and trying to get it over with as fast as she can. Having unwanted sex creates anger, distrust and resentment, and may end up cultivating an outright aversion to sex in the lower-libido partner. (Most often, it's the male partner who wants more sex, although sometimes the reverse is true.)

Some men feel as though they *need* to ejaculate daily. They may feel that the only acceptable way to achieve this is through intercourse. Most women are unlikely to want to keep up this pace, especially in midlife and beyond. Sex that is a purely a vehicle for ejaculation is usually brief and rarely satisfies the female partner in any significant way—by the time she's really ready, it's over. A man with this need can find other ways to address it besides intercourse. He can masturbate either by himself or in the presence of his partner (the latter, without asking her to get involved beyond kind, loving attention). If she wants to help him satisfy his need, she can do so with oral sex or by giving him a hand job (bringing him to orgasm with a lubricated hand). Couples who have this dynamic should be careful to communicate as openly and honestly as possible. The female partner should only "help out" when she truly wants to.

181

Keeping It Real

Sometimes, when date night rolls around, you might choose to go all-out to make it fun and super-sexy: get a bikini wax, buy some lingerie, watch an erotic movie or read a book about different positions in preparation for wowing your partner with a new technique or two. For the date itself, you might rent a sexy movie, get the kids set up for sleepovers, and make the bedroom romantic. Relax in a hot bath, and dream up new ways to have fun with your partner.

Other times, you might not want to prepare much at all. You might show up feeling rotten, having been able to do little to prepare besides brushing your teeth and taking a few deep breaths to try to release the tension of the day. If this is the case, that's what you and your partner need to make space for and communicate about. There's no requirement that you show up at your absolute sexiest and best for a date, and you don't have to do anything you really don't want to do. Your partner wants to connect with the real you, not with an act.

Bring whatever is real to your time together. Share your true feelings, communicate clearly and without blaming, and surprising things can happen.

What if, on the day of the date, the idea of sex ranks somewhere below dental surgery? What if you and your partner are having a fight, or if you just aren't feeling up to it? Go back to the awareness techniques in Chapter 8. Other techniques and tips given in this chapter will help as well.

Don't feel like you have to have intercourse during your date. You might use the time to find ways to reconnect on an intimate level. You might opt for "outercourse" —touching, caressing, holding, and other forms of giving and receiving pleasure. If one partner can't get him or herself in the mood no matter what, the other partner might masturbate while being lovingly held or watched, or the less sexed-up partner might give the other a hand job or oral sex. It's all good—as long as you both go there with the intention of creating and cultivating a satisfying intimate connection. The reason for the date is to experience pleasure together. It's an opportunity to give and receive appreciation and love.

One patient shared a story with me about this. She had an awful afternoon locked in power struggles with her young children. Her husband came home from work late and found her disheveled and cranky. "Our date tonight should be interesting," he said to her as she wrestled a toddler into his bath. She snapped at him but didn't cancel—even when he didn't offer to help. Then, when the kids were finally tucked away, all she wanted to do was yell at her husband, eat half a pint of ice cream, watch some brainless TV and pass out, but she didn't. She and her husband met in their bedroom for their date.

He had turned down the bed and lit some candles. Right away, she began to feel more relaxed, but before she could connect with him on any intimate level, she had to tell him how angry she was that he hadn't helped her out more that night. He had to hear her anger without defending himself. After apologizing, he told her a little about his hard day at work and explained that he hadn't seen how much she needed his help. They ended up feeling close and loving, but she still felt wound up and not present in her body.

They moved to the bed, and when he touched her softly she burst into tears. She let herself cry and release the stress of the day, and he held her without trying to get her to stop and let go of his own tension. As she calmed she focused on her breathing and they stroked each other. The sex that followed was brief but wonderfully intimate. They had spent most of their date time finding their way to a place where that could happen.

Moms: It's Okay To Insist on Privacy

Many moms are unwilling to tell the kids straight up that Mom and Dad are having alone time and that they should not interrupt. It can seem embarrassing, a case of "too much information" for kids who don't even want to *think* about what Mom and Dad might be doing in there with the door locked. Or mother-guilt raises its head; she thinks, *What if they need me and I'm not right there for them?*

To those moms: it's okay to lock the door to your bedroom when you and your husband want to be alone together—or, at the very least, to close it and to tell the children that they must knock if they need you. It's okay to sit the kids down and say, "If our bedroom door is closed, please do not knock or call out for us unless it's an emergency!" If they want to know what you're up to, just tell them, "We want to have some time alone together."

Of course, this doesn't apply if you have infants, toddlers or preschoolers. Children in these age groups need to be monitored constantly during their waking hours and often wake up at night. Sex can seem almost impossible for mothers of children this young when those children are in the house with her. This is especially true of parents who either co-sleep (sleep with babies or toddlers in the parents' bed) or have a child sleeping in a crib in their bedroom. Most mothers who sleep with or near their babies will have virtually no libido as long as that baby is near.

Nursing presents a unique libido challenge. It affects hormones in a way that can strongly reduce desire—and it's not a good idea to try to change those hormone levels as long as nursing continues. With more and more women opting to nurse babies for one or more years after they are born, this is not an insignificant concern. *I'll address it in more depth in Chapter 11.*

When children are younger than elementary age, it may be best to schedule date times when the kids are out of the house, at preschool or with a babysitter. You might try arranging a kid swap with like-minded friends: they take your children for your date time, and you return the favor. If you do co-sleep and want to have intimate time while your child sleeps in your bed, create another place in your house where you and your partner can have your dates.

If You're Postmenopausal and Haven't Had Sex In a Long Time

Women who are in menopause and have not had sex for months or years may experience considerable vaginal shrinking and dryness. Trying to have intercourse before restoring the tissues of the vagina and vulva with appropriate bioidentical hormone replacement therapy can be painful.

I advise postmenopausal patients who are returning to sex after a long break to give their BHRT a chance to plump out the tissues of the vagina and vulva before having intercourse. This takes, on average, four to six weeks. Trying to have intercourse or even to insert toys or fingers before the full effect of BHRT has kicked in may cause pain or even tear the vagina, which can then lead to involuntary vaginal contractions *(vaginismus)* that may make sex painful even after the hormones have taken effect. If any sexual activity is tried before this four-to-six-week point, be sure to use plenty of lubricant.

Once those four to six weeks have passed, I recommend starting to open and stretch the vagina with a generously lubricated finger (the woman's own or her partner's). The vaginal weights mentioned later in this chapter can also be used to gently stretch the vagina over time.

Enhancing Desire and Sensation

Women who aren't comfortable expressing their sexual desires may find it hard to imagine themselves trying some of the techniques suggested in the rest of this chapter. Depending on the generation in which they were born, the part of the world they're from, and their family, cultural and religious backgrounds, women have different levels of tolerance for going 'outside the box' of what's comfortable for them, especially in the realm of sexual desire. However, research shows that when couples take risks together and venture outside their usual comfort zones, their neurotransmitters change in ways that promote greater connectedness. Some sex therapists recommend that partners commit to do something new at each date to enhance intimacy.

As you venture into this new realm, keep in mind the communication pointers in Chapter 12. For a person who is not accustomed taking risks, it can be devastating to have a request or a suggestion slammed or laughed at by a partner. Be as receptive and sensitive as possible, even to ideas that seem too wild to follow through on.

Being adventurous doesn't have to involve being tied up or learning to pole dance. The new things you try can be subtle: giving each other a massage, maybe, or buying a cute nightie to surprise him on date night. Perhaps you could take turns blindfolding each other and feeding each other sensual foods like chocolate-covered strawberries. Try a new sexual position. Surprise your partner with a racy card game or board game.

You never have to try something new if you don't want to do, but there's no harm in fully listening to your partner's suggestion. If it's too much for you, perhaps there's a modified version that would spice up your love life.

Awareness, blood flow and energy

Now that time for sex is on the calendar, I'd like to suggest a few exercises that will bring awareness, blood flow, and energy to your organs of desire.

First, just practice these exercises on your own, separate from being sexual. Use them to cultivate awareness of your body and to rediscover your sensual self. Then, you can bring that awareness into masturbation; and then, when you are comfortable with that awareness as a part of your sexuality, bring it into sex with your partner.

Kegel Exercises. Kegels (pronounced "KAY-gulls") are strength training exercises for the vagina and the muscles that support the pelvic organs (uterus, bladder and ovaries). They involve rhythmically contracting and releasing the *pubococcygeus* (PC) muscles.

Kegels don't actually *tighten* the vagina, but they do build the muscles around the vagina, giving you a greater ability to contract your vagina, which can be very exciting for your partner! Kegels increase blood flow to the vagina and clitoris, which enhances the ability to become sexually aroused.

Kegels also help prevent uterine prolapse and control urinary incontinence, which is fairly common in women from midlife forward—especially those who have given birth.

Here's how to do a Kegel exercise: the next time you urinate, try to stop mid-stream without contracting the muscles of your buttocks, thighs or abdomen. Now you know what Kegels feel like. The muscles that accomplish this are your PC muscles.

To strengthen and tone the PC muscles, work up to doing ten to 20 Kegels two or three times a day, holding the PC muscles in their contracted position for two to ten seconds. They don't always have to be held; vary the pattern by doing them fast, slow and rhythmically. Kegels can be done anywhere—sitting in traffic, sitting at your desk, or standing in line.

Doing a set of Kegels just before a date will enhance blood flow to your vagina, and a consistent practice will enhance the contractions that occur during orgasm. (Kegels can also be done by men to promote arousal and better genital blood flow.) They can also be done during sex or masturbation to intensify sensation. If you do them while your partner's penis is inside you, it will feel to him as though you're massaging him with the walls of your vagina. Vaginal weights, which are inserted into the vagina and held there while doing Kegels, can be purchased online or in stores that sell sex toys.

Libido strengthening and warm-up exercises

The exercises and tips listed below can be done on an ongoing basis or can be used as lead-ins to sex. They can be done in the half hour or 20 minutes before you meet up for your date, or they can be brought back during sex if you feel the need to re-ground into your body and your sensations. All of these exercises can be done with your partner during your time together.

In Chapter 8 you learned about using mindfulness as a tool for becoming more aware and present in your body. Here, we'll focus on exercises that specifically enhance libido and sensual experience.

Pamper yourself before a date. Take time before a date to pamper yourself and tune in to your sensual nature. Eat something delicious, then take a warm bath with bubbles or a few drops of an aromatic oil. Smooth on naturally scented body oil or lotion (try making your own, combining cold-pressed almond oil with a few drops of an organic essential oil such as lavender, patchouli, jasmine, rose, sandalwood or musk), taking time to massage it into every inch of your skin.

Conscious breathing can increase arousal and spread sexual energy throughout the body. Practices that consciously cultivate sexual energy throughout the body will help bring back pleasure and intimacy in a relationship that hasn't been sexual for awhile—or that hasn't been sexually satisfying despite the efforts of both partners. It can also help men and women shift from work/parent consciousness to sensuality and intimacy.

David Deida is a teacher and author who specializes in helping both men and women to merge the sexual and the spiritual. In his book, *The Enlightened Sex Manual: Sexual Skills for the Superior Lover* (Sounds True, 2007), he gives helpful pointers for using breath to circulate sexual energy and relax into desire.

Deida explains that in conscious breathing, the inhalation is an opening to receive from your partner. The exhalation is a release of tension, which allows you to experience more love and pleasure and to enjoy giving to your partner.

Inhalation brings energy to the genitals. To do this, imagine inhalations moving down the front of your body, through the area of the belly, and filling the belly and sexual organs with energy.

Exhalation releases energy. Deida describes the exhaled breath as "a form of surrender." If you tend to be tense, easily angered or anxious, Deida says, you are probably not fully exhaling, and will benefit from consciously trying to deepen and lengthen your exhalations. He also mentions that men who tend to ejaculate prematurely tend to be shallow exhalers, as are women who can orgasm easily but who never feel like their orgasms are very powerful.

Cultivate Your Own Garden First. Some women who find themselves disappointed with or turned off by sex want to blame their partners. Perhaps he isn't very skilled in bed; perhaps he has issues with premature ejaculation or ejaculatory dysfunction; maybe he just isn't all that interested in giving pleasure to his partner.

Regardless of the shortcomings of your partner, the way back to an enlivened libido and satisfying sex life comes first through cultivating sexual energy and libido in yourself. Take control of your own sexuality—and then, when you bring it to your partner, you'll be clear about what you want, and you can work on communicating this to him. By doing the practices described in this chapter, you are taking responsibility for your own sexual pleasure and satisfaction. To put it another way: you're tuning your instrument perfectly and practicing thoroughly before you go to play with your duet partner.

Masturbation: Lovemaking for one

When I ask patients whether they masturbate, I get all kinds of answers. Some women are simply not interested in touching themselves "down

189

there." Others have a lot of experience with pleasuring themselves, and this is one of the things they miss doing once their libidos wane.

Masturbation can be most beneficial for women who have not had sex in a long time and who don't yet feel comfortable going there with a partner. It is also helpful for women who find it difficult to remain present and aware during sex with their partners, who don't have as much sensation as they'd like, or who have difficulty reaching orgasm during sex.

Masturbation can contribute a lot to a monogamous sexual relationship— particularly when approached as a slow, sensual, aware process where you learn all there is to know about your own body and how it experiences the most pleasure. It provides a safe space to practice being at heightened levels of sexual pleasure while remaining relaxed and aware.

Either before a date or on a non-date occasion, get comfortable in a private place. Light a candle and wear sexy lingerie or whatever else helps you feel your most beautiful. Use your own hands to explore all of your non-genital and genital erogenous zones. Try fantasizing, watching a sexy movie, reading erotica or looking at erotic art while you masturbate.

Breathe deeply and follow your instincts. If self-consciousness comes up, just "fake it till you make it"—a good practice for letting your guard down with your partner. Whatever you choose to do during this time, and however long you choose to do it, the point isn't to reach any goal—it's to get comfortable with being sexual, and to bring your awareness and intention to sexual sensation and pleasure. Anything you do solo, you can do with your partner. Chances are good that your partner would love to watch you masturbate.

What about sex toys?

I get diverse reactions from patients about sex toys, too. Some women cringe at the idea of using a vibrator or dildo. Other women tell me that in their sexier days, they were enthusiastic collectors and users of sex toys.

For the uninitiated, here's a brief rundown of toys to consider trying. Most can be purchased at novelty stores, but these days, the best place to shop for these items is on the Internet. Try Good Vibrations (**www.goodvibrations.com**) or Adam & Eve (**www.adameve.com**) for starters.

Vibrators

Vibrators have been around since the 1880s, when they were developed to spare physicians the responsibility of giving vulvar and clitoral massages to women who had been diagnosed with "hysteria." Bringing these women to orgasm seemed to cure them, but doing it by hand was hard work.

Vibrators are helpful for women who are challenged with reaching orgasm. When held against the clitoris, anus or vulva, they can bring on intense orgasms. Many types are available. Choose sex toys that are phthalate-free— free of the carcinogenic, estrogenic chemicals found in some plastics. Some vibrators plug into the wall; others are battery-operated.

- Clitoral vibrators can be wand-shaped with a handle or small and button-shaped (the latter may be called a "pocket rocket;" small vibrators that look like lipsticks, cell phones or other small objects are also available). They are held against the clitoris but aren't meant for vaginal penetration. (These are also sold as general massagers.)

- Rabbit vibrators (also known as "jackrabbits") have a long, penis-like part and a small extension on one side that can be used to stimulate the clitoris. They may be made of latex, polyvinyl chloride, silicone or rubber. The shafts of many jackrabbit vibrators rotate and have textured surfaces.

- Dildo-shaped vibrators have a vibrating tip and have a long shape that can be used for vaginal penetration. These do double duty as dildoes (see below) and vibrators. They may be made of vinyl, latex or silicone.

- G-spot vibrators are similar to dildo-shaped vibrators, but with a significant difference: they're curved to make G-spot stimulation easier.

- Love eggs are egg-shaped vibrators that can be inserted completely into the vagina. They may be made of metal, glass, plastic or composite materials.

- Butterfly vibrators are shaped like butterflies and come with straps that allow them to be used hands-free. They can be used during intercourse.

- Men can wear what's known as a cock ring—a ring that goes around the base of the penis to create and maintain a harder, fuller erection—that is fitted with a small vibrator. During intercourse, the vibrator stimulates the woman's clitoris.

Textured surfaces on vibrators and dildoes can increase sensation for the user.

Dildoes

These are basically penis substitutes. Some are lifelike stand-alone penises made of silicone, plastic or rubber. Dildoes can also be made of wood, glass or other materials. They've been in use since prehistoric times—in those days, dildoes were carved out of stone. Men with erectile dysfunction or who tend to ejaculate prematurely can use dildoes (or vibrators) to help satisfy their partners when their own bodies are less than cooperative.

All of these toys are best paired with a water-based lubricant. Have a lubricant handy for dates, as well. I often prescribe Scream Cream, a vaginal lubricant that contains the amino acid arginine to dilate vulvar and vaginal blood vessels and increase arousal. K*Y makes a lubricant that contains niacin, a B vitamin, which also has the effect of increasing blood flow and arousal, and mint, which enhances sensation.

Many other objects can be used to enhance masturbation or sex. Feathers, fur, sensuous fabrics, ice, lotions, massagers, massage oils, blindfolds, pleasing scents, sensual music, special lingerie and other props can all be kept in the same place as sex toys, erotica or pornography, should you choose to use them. Keep your box hidden away and bring it out when date time comes along.

Erotica, pornography and fantasy

Erotica can come in the form of books, online content or magazines. It can be written or visual, and it doesn't have to be trashy or lowbrow! It's important to avoid pornography that is demeaning to either men or women. There are many wonderful books of erotic art that include sexually explicit paintings and drawings by some of history's most renowned artists. Browse the Erotica section in your local bookstore or at an online bookseller to find titles that help awaken your libido. Or purchase an illustrated how-to book or card deck that includes explicit drawings or photographs of couples making love in lots of different positions.

Web bookseller Abe Books' list of the sexiest literature of all time includes:

John Cleland's Fanny Hill: *Memoirs of a Woman of Pleasure*
D.H. Lawrence's *Lady Chatterley's Lover*
Henry Miller's *Tropic of Cancer*
Pauline Reage's *Story of O*
J.G. Ballard's *Crash*
Philip Roth's *Portnoy's Complaint*
Erica Jong's *Fear of Flying*
Anne Rice's *Interview With the Vampire*
Susan Minot's *Raptures*
A.M. Homes' *The End of Alice*

The memoirs of Catherine Millet, Toni Bentley, Elizabeth McNeill, Emmanuelle Arsan, Frank Harris and Hedy Lamarr made Playboy's top 10 list of sexiest American memoirs. Some women love romance novels; others enjoy reading pornographic *Penthouse* Forum letters! Find what arouses you and enjoy it.

Pornography has less than positive connotations for many women. It's an especially touchy issue for women whose partners have gotten caught up in a private relationship with Internet porn. It can feel as though your partner is cheating on you with a long line of young, hot girls who want nothing more than to take off their clothes and give pleasure.

However, pornography can bring excitement and desire to both partners when used as a supplement to a monogamous sex life—as long as both partners are comfortable with what's being used, and as long as it's not used as a distraction from or replacement for actual intimacy between partners. A lot of pornography is just plain boring, particularly for women—just scene after scene of people having intercourse very, very close up. It may take some searching to find videos that you and your partner will both enjoy. Pornography that is demeaning or abusive will not enhance libido or intimacy in a healthy relationship.

Instructional sex videos can be just as arousing as porn films—and they teach you something in the bargain! For detailed sexual how-tos, including instruction on Tantric sex, try one or more of the wonderful books, videos and classes available.

Never before have couples had this much access to great erotica, sex information and education, and sex toys. Most everything can ordered on the internet, so there's no worry about being embarrassed in the library or bookstore checkout line, or having to browse a novelty store. Once you decide to get on the road back to a satisfying sex life, there's virtually no limit to what you can learn and try.

PART III

The Ages and Cycles of Sexuality and Libido

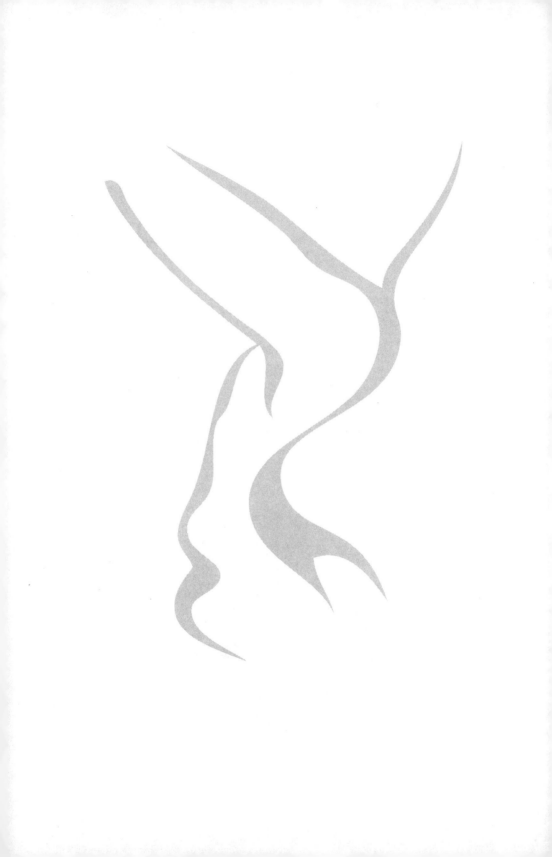

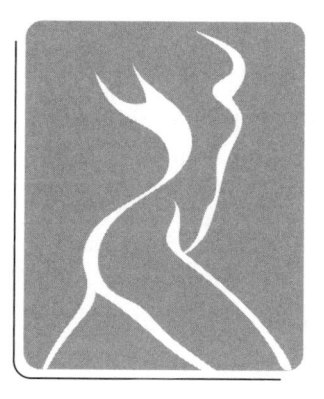

CHAPTER 11

Childbirth and Children

Flirting, sexual attraction, desire and sexual pleasure are all part of nature's design to lure us into reproducing. But then, once the baby arrives, sex tends to fall way to the bottom of the priority list.

From here, the story's pretty predictable. Once she recovers from giving birth, Mom feels overwhelmed with the responsibilities of new motherhood. She isn't sleeping well. Most of her waking hours are spent holding her baby. If she's nursing, she's probably coping with engorged breasts, leaking milk and the grind of constant breastfeeding. Sometimes she doesn't even have a chance to shower or eat an uninterrupted meal. The lumpy sweats she throws on every morning don't help her forget the way her body has changed with this pregnancy. On top of this, she is usually the one who does the household chores, cooks and cares for older children.

And then this man who disappears all day comes home to eat the meal she's cooked and spends ten minutes helping out with the kids before bedtime wants to *what*? When Mom finally has a few minutes of peace? He wants to touch her just when she gets a reprieve from constant touching? At this point, all Mom can think about is getting as much sleep as possible before the baby wakes up for a feeding. Dad is going to have to take care of himself. Again.

Mom's estrogen and progesterone levels are low for weeks (if she formula-feeds) to months (if she breastfeeds) after giving birth, and this strongly impacts her libido. A new mother tends to be so filled with the experience of mothering her new baby that she doesn't miss having sex with her partner. Her partner—who, if he's like most men, hasn't experienced any drop in sex drive since becoming a father, regardless of the changes in her body that make her feel anything but sexual—ends up feeling as though this tiny new person has completely displaced him in his partner's life. If he dares to express any hint of resentment, he might find himself on the receiving end of a furious tirade about how she has to do everything around here and he just doesn't understand how exhausted she is. Out of guilt or obligation, she might submit to his advances once in a while, but he knows she's not into it, and that's no fun for him.

Eventually the man might give up on trying to initiate sex with his wife because she seems too busy being a mother. He gets tired of being rejected. Both partners begin to think that a healthy sex life and parenthood just can't coexist. Maybe they'll start having sex again and enjoying it once the kids are a little older. Or maybe when they start school...or when they leave for college.

So many couples are unprepared for this shift. In the worst cases, it can create a rift between partners that can only be mended with lots of counseling, or that can lead to infidelity and divorce. If you're at a place in your life where you need to reconcile your mommy self with the self that has satisfying sex, this chapter should help you to navigate the obstacles parenthood can create to a healthy libido.

The First Few Months

During my residency, I suffered through the standard ordeal of 80- to 100-hour weeks, working for days with very little sleep. It was a breeze compared to being the mother of infants less than six months old.

For the first six months of a baby's life, a new mom should not feel obligated to work on her libido. All of her time and effort will be focused on caring for the new arrival and any other children who are already part of the family. When she's not doing this, she needs to sleep. This being said, women should definitely not have any kind of penetrative sex before six to eight weeks after giving birth. The uterus needs to shrink back to its pre-pregnancy size before sex resumes; otherwise there is a risk of infection. Women who experience tearing or have episiotomies during childbirth will require at least this much time to heal before they can have sex without pain.

It takes up to a year for a woman's hormones to return to their normal cycles and levels following the birth of a child. This will happen more slowly in women who breastfeed than in those who formula feed (more on this below). My usual advice is to start thinking about returning to a regular sexual connection once the first six months or so have passed.

Overwhelming fatigue is the usual first barrier. A mom who hasn't gotten a full night's sleep for months is likely to choose sleep over sex for as long as the baby continues to awaken several times each night. Some parents and experts deal with this through sleep training, using techniques like those created by Dr. Richard Ferber.

"Ferberizing" can start at about four to six months of age. Parents are instructed to engage the baby in a loving, consistent bedtime routine, and then to put the baby down in her crib while she's still awake. In response to any crying, the parents go in and briefly comfort the baby without picking her up or feeding her. As the sleep training progresses, the baby is left to cry for longer and longer periods. Ideally, the baby learns to soothe herself to sleep over the course of a few days of Ferberizing.

Other parents choose co-sleeping (where the baby is kept near or in the parents' bed to make nighttime feedings and soothing less disruptive to the parents' sleep). Moms who co-sleep can nurse their babies without getting out of bed, and they may find that they get a lot more sleep this way. Co-sleepers, which are modified cribs that attach to an adult bed, can keep baby within arm's reach but out of the parents' bed.

Some mothers catch up on sleep when the baby sleeps (going to bed early and napping with the baby during the day so that disrupted sleep doesn't have as strong an impact), or they may share nighttime feeding and changing responsibilities with Dad.

One question that often comes up about co-sleeping (also known as "the family bed"): when your bed has a baby in it, where do Mom and Dad go to have sex? A sleeping infant who's on one side of a big bed or in a co-sleeper or crib in the parents' room isn't likely to be disturbed when her parents make love nearby, as long as they're quiet and not too acrobatic. If they would rather be alone, parents who sleep with their children can create a separate area in the house where they go to have sex.

Whatever route you choose, if your baby is six months old and you're still feeling completely sleep-deprived, take action to try to improve the situation before you focus on resurrecting your sex life!

Breastfeeding and post-partum libido

A woman about to give birth has estrogen and progesterone levels hundreds of times greater than a non-pregnant, regularly cycling woman. As soon as the baby is born, levels of both hormones plummet.

If the new mom breastfeeds, levels of another hormone, *prolactin*, rise. Prolactin stimulates the milk glands to produce milk. Every time the baby feeds, another surge of prolactin comes from the pituitary gland (a small gland located at the base of the brain) into the bloodstream. Prolactin suppresses production of *gonadotropin releasing hormone*, or GnRH, the hormone that stimulates estrogen and progesterone production in the ovaries. As long as nursing provides the baby's main source of nourishment, prolactin will stay high and estrogen and progesterone will remain low.

Whether the hormones of libido drop during lactation or menopause, the results are similar: vaginal dryness, thinning of the vaginal wall, and less arousal in response to stimulation. Without plenty of lubricant, intercourse can be painful for a woman who is breastfeeding. Bioidentical hormone replacement isn't an option for nursing mothers. Raising levels of progesterone or estrogens during lactation could interfere with milk production, and hormones could pass into breast milk.

In a nursing mother, breasts and nipples become super-sensitive, and any stimulation of these areas can cause milk to let down or leak. Orgasm can cause milk to leak or even spurt. (While some couples don't find this bothersome during lovemaking, women who would rather keep breast milk and sex separate may want to wear a bra with nursing pads inside during sex.) Some women can easily experience their breasts as both feeding stations and erogenous zones; others clearly don't want their partner to go anywhere near their nipples once their breasts have been through months or years of nursing babies.

Oxytocin, the "cuddle hormone," which is produced during orgasm and physical closeness with a partner, is also responsible for ejection of milk from the breast. Some nursing mothers become more turned off to sex because of concerns that nursing and sexual arousal are linked. It's rare that a woman actually becomes aroused while breastfeeding, but in our culture—where female breasts are primarily thought of as sexual, not as protrusions designed to feed babies—this concern comes up fairly often. It can sometimes cause new mothers to stop nursing… or it can boot sex even further down the priority list for as long as breastfeeding continues.

Although nursing for a year is best for your baby, the fact is that many mothers stop much sooner, for a long list of reasons—which may include needing to get her body back and to focus more on intimacy with her partner. Many women feel undue pressure to keep breastfeeding even when it's causing their lives to fall out of balance or when it's physically uncomfortable or painful for them. A happy mother with a balanced life is just as good for her baby as breast milk. Weaning will restore hormonal cycles that create libido.

Any woman who has breast-fed knows that it changes the shape and firmness of the breasts. The longer she breastfeeds, the more pronounced these changes are likely to be. This can be challenging when a woman's breasts have been a major turn-on to her partner in the past, but breastfeeding's benefits to your baby and to you (it reduces your risk of breast and ovarian cancers) are worth a little sagging!

Mommies Don't Have Sex, Do They?

On a daytime talk show a sex therapist talked to a series of married couples about the loss of their sexual connection. One woman shared that even the thought of being sexual with her husband made her feel like she was neglecting or betraying her children. Their marriage was falling apart, but she felt she had to choose her children over her husband—what good mom wouldn't?

The camera panned out over the audience, showing many other women nodding their heads. This problem obviously struck a chord.

It's completely natural to not even think about sex for the first six months of a new baby's life. Hormonal shifts, exhaustion, trauma from difficult births or other biological changes explain much of the drop in libido most women experience in those first few weeks to months after giving birth. It can take a year for libido to come back on its own. There are other reasons for this drop in libido—like the belief that moms don't do that naughty stuff—that can be shifted.

If the last time you remember having a libido was before you became a mother, and if this has gone on for more than six months, consider whether you believe that cultivating a sex life with your husband means that you aren't doing what you need to be doing for your kids. Do you find yourself distracted from your partner and his needs by a constantly running mental checklist of your child or children's needs?

"My kids are always on my mind...*always*," said one patient. "When I go to bed with my husband and he starts wanting to touch and kiss me, that doesn't change. Even when they're sleeping, I'm aware of their presence in the next room. And thinking about my kids makes it impossible for me to get in the mood for sex. It just feels wrong." Many women feel as though motherhood interferes with their libidos for years after their children are born.

American culture has created a steep divide between motherhood and sexuality. Being sexy has come to conflict directly with being maternal. This cultural subtext tells women that putting time and energy into staying sexy and having a satisfying sex life means that they are less fit as mothers.

Besides: devoting time and effort to hair, makeup or clothes might seem ludicrous to the mom who only leaves the house to grocery shop and take the toddler to a doctor's appointment! Out come the mommy haircuts and sweats; away go the cute outfits and tasteful makeup palettes that once made her feel sexy.

The simple awareness that this internal battle of mommy self vs. sexual partner self is going on can help in the understanding that you can devote some of your energy toward cultivating a healthy sex life without compromising yourself as a mother. Sexual intimacy is important for creating harmony in most marriages, and you and your partner are responsible for setting the example for your children in terms of what a loving relationship looks and feels like.

What About Contraception?

Once you're back to having sex, avoid using oral contraceptives, patches or the Mirena IUD (an intrauterine device that delivers progestins daily to the lining of the uterus) while nursing. Hormonal contraceptives reduce libido, primarily by reducing testosterone levels. Some studies suggest that it is unsafe to expose breastfeeding infants to progestins in mother's milk.

Progestins are bad for libido, period. They suppress the production of follicle stimulating hormone (which causes an egg to ripen in the ovary each month) and luteinizing hormone (which stimulates the release of the egg and the surge of progesterone that follows it). Measurements of estrogen and progesterone in a woman using this type of contraception can look like those of a woman in menopause! Use barrier methods (keep in mind that cervical caps and diaphragms may need to be re-sized after giving birth) or a Paragard IUD (the type that does not use hormones).

Although on-demand exclusive breastfeeding does suppress ovulation, I don't recommend using it as a birth control method! You can conceive again even before you have that first post-partum period.

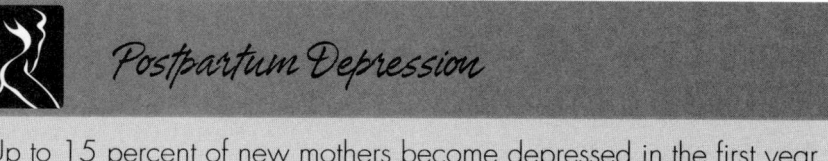

Postpartum Depression

Up to 15 percent of new mothers become depressed in the first year or two after giving birth. For the mom who is extremely sad, can't sleep, has no energy, and feels she can't bond with her baby, rekindling libido can wait. She needs help to feel like herself again.

The usual treatment for postpartum depression (PPD) is an antidepressant — most often, for nursing mothers, the drug of choice is Zoloft because less of it passes into breast milk than other antidepressants. Antidepressants often suppress libido. Non-drug interventions can work, too: family and friends can pitch in to help Mom get enough sleep and have an hour a day to relax with no responsibilities. Light therapy (sitting near a small light that emits the same kind of radiation as the sun for a period of time each day — especially helpful in northern latitudes or where it's often cloudy or rainy, or in winter when days are shorter), counseling and exercise have also been found helpful for postpartum depression.

There's some evidence that hormonal imbalances play a role in postpartum depression in a subgroup of women who develop it. Women who are no longer nursing may find that hormone balancing with bioidenticals helps to relieve their PPD symptoms. The woman whose depression feels anxious and agitated may be estrogen dominant, especially if she has other symptoms of estrogen dominance, in which case antidepressants may not work. Natural progesterone may be just what's needed.

How To Renew Your Sex Life Post-Partum

Set the intention to re-kindle the fires that resulted in those adorable children. Find a way to get enough sleep. Then, follow the advice in other chapters about cultivating mindfulness, setting a schedule, keeping your sex life interesting and varied, and working through relationship issues.

Make time to be together one-on-one. Go on dates and leave the kids with a family member or sitter; if money for a sitter is an issue, arrange child-care swaps with another family so that you all get to have time away from the kids to re-connect and remember why you love being together.

You're so much more than a mom. Remember all the things that used to excite you before you had kids? Keep them a part of your life, even if it's just a fraction of what it used to be. Enthusiasm and curiosity make everything better, including your sex life. Remind your partner of all that you are. Insist that he treat you as more than a mom, too!

If that includes helping you out with more of the chores and taking over the child-care duties once in a while, so be it. Tell your partner clearly how he can help you maintain the mental space and energy necessary for sex. "Honey, I know we have our date tonight," you might tell him after dinner. "I could use some time to freshen up, so I'll need you to take care of the dishes and get the kids ready for bed." Pat him on the behind, kiss him on the cheek, tell him how much you love and appreciate him, and head for the tub.

Some moms can get a little control-freaky over the way things need to be done in their households. The dishes have to be done just so; the laundry, ditto; the children need this particular food or to have their routines carried out in exactly Mom's way. While a little control-freakiness can be enormously helpful in keeping a busy household running smoothly, some moms end up not delegating any of the work to their partners because, in her opinion, the guy just doesn't do any of it right!

If this describes you, I'd suggest letting go enough to realize that even if Dad mixes the lights and the darks or if he doesn't get the dishes sparkling clean like you do; even if he sends the 8 year old to bed without a shower or feeds the toddler ice cream while you aren't watching—it's okay. Take a deep breath and be grateful that you have a partner who's willing to help out in his own way. Look for all he's doing right and verbally express your appreciation. When you look back years from now, you won't cherish clean dishes or the properly folded shirts nearly as much as you'll appreciate the results of the time and effort spent cultivating a loving relationship with your partner.

Giving birth changes things...Down there and all over

A vaginal birth stretches the vagina to its limits and may cause tearing or "skid marks" (extreme stretching). Episiotomies are often performed in an attempt to prevent tearing. The whole process of pregnancy and birth can alter the look and sensation of the vagina and vulva. When you first start to make dates with your partner, take some time to explore these changes and get comfortable with them. Have your partner touch and explore you gently to get used to the new you. If your partner saw you give birth, he may need some time to get used to seeing that part of you the way he once did. Women who had traumatic experiences giving birth or who required a C-section may need even more time and care to feel sexual again. Let this exploration and sensual touching phase go on until you feel comfortable and safe.

A postpartum body that's heavier than it once was or has a more stretched-out belly can bring feelings of self-consciousness. It's easy to think, "When I lose this baby weight, *then* we can start having sex again." Eat well and exercise, and then accept that this is the body you're in at the moment. It's the body your partner wants to have sex with! Take good care of your skin, keep your hair cut and clean, and put on some nice clothes once in a while. Make and keep your dates and cultivate sexual energy using the techniques described in previous chapters.

Having a great sex life doesn't depend on the look of your breasts or your belly; it's about pleasure and connection. Couples who thoroughly enjoy each other sexually make happier, healthier, more balanced parents. Don't let a few extra pounds or stretch marks stand in the way of that.

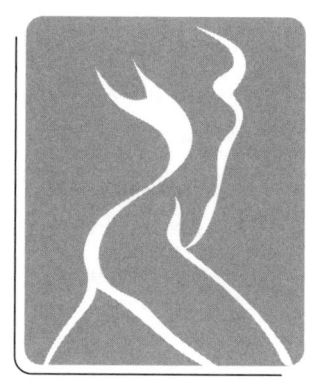

CHAPTER 12

The Fluctuating Forties

Since entering her 40s, Ingrid had been troubled by low libido, weight gain and fatigue. Her own research had convinced her that hormone imbalances were the most likely reason for these issues. She and I worked together for almost three years to bring her hormones into balance. As her 40-something husband watched Ingrid become healthier, he began to see me for the same reasons! This couple was strongly motivated to be their healthiest selves during this decade of life.

Ingrid went from being 30 pounds overweight, exhausted all the time, out of shape and mildly depressed to being a slim, strong athlete—she even trained for and walked in an event where competitors cover one and a half marathons' worth of ground over a period of two days! Her husband couldn't keep up with her on the fitness front, as he had a high-stress job that involved frequent travel, but he was feeling a lot better. He was very happy that his libido had returned.

Although Ingrid's hormones and her life seemed to have come into good balance, one important piece of the puzzle still refused to fall into place: her libido. On a day when we took some time to discuss this during an appointment, she said, "I realized something lately. I'm very visual—I make sense of the world through my eyes, what I see. And recently…well, I'll just come out and say it. I'm not liking the visual with my husband."

"Your husband's body, you mean?" I asked. "It's not arousing for you to look at?"

"Right! The feel is good. The visual is not."

We talked for a while about how she might adapt to this—aside from nagging her husband to work out more to get rid of his spare tire. I encouraged her to develop her other senses in lovemaking: scent, sound, feel. "Find music that helps you get in the mood. Focus on how good he feels and on how much you love him." I also suggested she look into erotica or try fantasy to help boost her libido.

Another patient, Joanna, showed up in my office with typical fourth-decade complaints. She and her husband Paul, at 47 and 63 respectively, with their teen sons nearly grown, wanted to renew their sexual spark. Paul responded almost immediately to hormones; his libido surged and his erections, which had not been terribly reliable before, were ready for action. He had recently retired and had plenty of energy for sex, but Joanna still wasn't feeling it, despite hormone balancing. Paul was starting to wonder whether she just found him undesirable. He had started to talk about divorce.

Finally, Joanna shared some details that I hadn't yet heard. Their sex life had gotten boring. "Why would I want to have sex three times a week in exactly the same boring missionary position with the lights out and my eyes closed?" she asked, exasperated. She was starved for novelty and felt like their sex life had hit a rut years ago, but Paul didn't see any problem with doing it the same way every time. In fact, he was resistant to trying anything new. Joanna resented Paul's new freedom as a retiree; she was consumed with the demands of her career, while still shouldering most of the work of running the household and caring for their sons. They spent much of their time together bickering over what seemed like petty stuff. It was obvious to me that this couple needed therapy.

Is It Your Hormones... or Is It Your Relationship?

Getting hormones in balance benefits overall health and libido, but if you're not feeling attracted to your partner, if you're too overwhelmed with work, or if your relationship is foundering, even the most skilled hormone balancing won't bring back that spark. Although it's easier to balance hormones than it is to fix an ailing relationship, the former won't compensate for the latter when it comes to rekindling libido.

Both kinds of issues—those having to do with hormones and those having to do with relationship—tend to bubble to the surface during a woman's fortieth decade. In most aspects of her life, she is finding her voice and her power in ways she never could before. At the same time, her hormones may be undergoing dramatic shifts.

Other concerns may come up in a woman's 40s. Some women have waited to have children or decide they want one more child after turning 40 but then struggle to conceive or have trouble carrying a pregnancy to term. Others have already had children and are wondering where their lives will go as their children need them less and less. Add these concerns to the hormonal roller-coaster many women find themselves on during these years, and it's no surprise that the 40s can be both incredibly fulfilling and incredibly challenging.

Judith Reichman, M.D., author of the book *I'm Not In the Mood: What Every Woman Should Know About Improving Her Libido* (William Morrow and Company 1998) points out that, "We often ignore relationship problems in our twenties and thirties, while we're raising our children, building our career and paying our mortgage. But once the children have left the home... our marital troubles can become magnified, sometimes to the point where we question the need for a relationship...Our relationship becomes a business partnership, where we share housekeeping, financial and social obligations, but not intimacy. We are too exhausted from our other pursuits to even think about sex. We get out of the habit and subsequently lose desire."

Later in this chapter, I'll share what I've learned about a specific form of relationship therapy that can help strengthen and renew the bond between partners—and offer a few specific pointers for husbands of women in their forties to help them get more of what they want in the bedroom. First, let's look at the ways in which hormones shift during a woman's 40s and the effect those shifts can have on health, well-being and libido.

Premenopause and Estrogen Dominance

The hormonal shifts that occur between a woman's mid-30s and early 50s are very different from those that occur right around the time of menopause. John Lee, M.D., who first popularized the use of bioidentical hormones, distinguished this stage of life from *perimenopause* by giving it a different name: *premenopause*. Perimenopause describes the year or two just before menopause, where estrogen, progesterone and testosterone all drop as periods come less frequently and then stop. Premenopause describes hormonal shifts that can begin in the mid-30s, as much as 20 years before menopause itself.

In the 20s and 30s, the hormonal cycles of most women run smoothly. Then, as early as a woman's mid-30s, hormonal shifts begin to take place. Some women begin to have *anovulatory* menstrual cycles—in which every few months the ovaries don't release an egg and no progesterone is produced to balance the effects of estrogen. Enough estrogen is produced to build up the uterine lining, and menstruation still occurs; but for that cycle, the ratio of estrogen to progesterone is skewed. This creates a state of *estrogen dominance.* Estrogen levels aren't necessarily too high and may even be below the optimum, but with the natural balancing effect of progesterone absent, estrogen's impact is greater. In addition, even ovulatory cycles tend to produce less progesterone. A woman who is estrogen dominant is more likely to experience worsening PMS, difficult or irregular periods, mood swings, mental fogginess, fat gain in the abdomen and hips, headaches, bloating, fluid retention, a chronically red face, anxiety, depression, fatigue and a sudden worsening of allergies, asthma, skin problems and sinus congestion.

Anovulatory cycles aren't the only factor in creating estrogen dominance. Being overweight or obese increases estrogen production (fat cells produce estrogens). Shifts in cortisol, insulin and adrenaline caused by chronic stress will also shift hormone balance in the direction of estrogen dominance.

Our environment is full of synthetic chemicals that act as estrogen mimics in the body. These chemicals are called *xenoestrogens* (which translates to "foreign estrogens") and are found in virtually every arena of modern life. Solvents, cleaning products, cosmetics, body care products, fragrances in air fresheners and fabric softeners, weed killers, sunscreens, insecticides, paints, dyes and building materials all contain these chemicals. Some have weak estrogenic effects, while some exert much stronger effects—strong enough to contribute to estrogen dominance, and sometimes even strong enough to be carcinogenic. We're all exposed to these chemicals, which add to our overall estrogen burden. Even men can become estrogen dominant from living in this soup of estrogenic pollutants.

Chronic stress and adrenal fatigue, which are discussed in depth in Chapter 8, are major causes of low progesterone levels in women in their 40s. Why? Cortisol and progesterone are both built from the same precursor: a hormone called pregnenolone. When cortisol production drops, the body will shunt more pregnenolone into cortisol production, which means less raw material for the building of progesterone. This makes perfect biological sense: if a woman's stress response system doesn't work properly, her body is in no condition to carry, bear, or care for a child. Low progesterone levels make conception much less likely while cortisol production is sub-par. For most women, returning to balance requires stress management.

Here is a more complete list of symptoms and conditions associated with estrogen dominance.

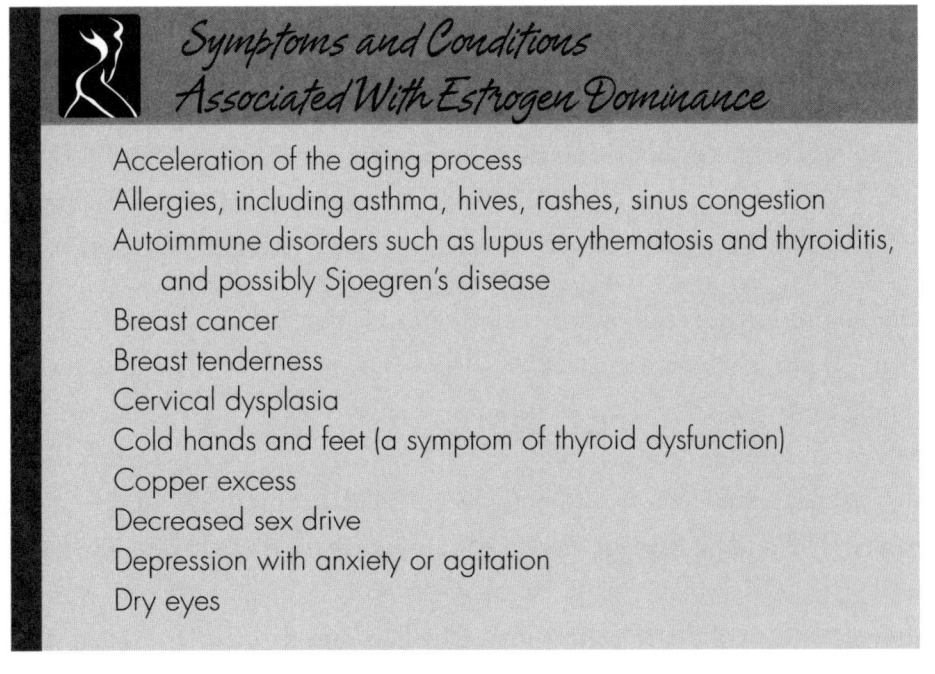

Symptoms and Conditions Associated With Estrogen Dominance

Acceleration of the aging process
Allergies, including asthma, hives, rashes, sinus congestion
Autoimmune disorders such as lupus erythematosis and thyroiditis, and possibly Sjoegren's disease
Breast cancer
Breast tenderness
Cervical dysplasia
Cold hands and feet (a symptom of thyroid dysfunction)
Copper excess
Decreased sex drive
Depression with anxiety or agitation
Dry eyes

Early onset of menstruation
Endometrial (uterine) cancer
Fat gain, especially around the abdomen, hips and thighs
Fatigue
Fibrocystic breasts
Foggy thinking
Gallbladder disease
Hair Loss
Headaches
Hypoglycemia
Increased blood clotting (increasing risk of strokes)
Infertility
Irregular menstrual periods
Irritability
Insomnia
Magnesium deficiency
Memory loss
Mood swings
Osteoporosis
Polycystic ovaries
Premenopausal bone loss
PMS
Sluggish metabolism
Thyroid dysfunction mimicking hypothyroidism
Uterine cancer
Uterine fibroids
Water retention, bloating
Zinc deficiency

(Reprinted with permission from *What Your Doctor May not Tell You About Menopause* by John R. Lee, MD and Virginia Hopkins)

Estrogen dominance, libido and the Pill

A woman who's feeling bloated, fat, blotchy, crampy, headachy, sore-breasted, moody and exhausted isn't going to want to have sex. She probably won't even want to show her body to her partner. The downward spiral might accelerate as she gives up on trying to keep her body fit or eating healthy foods. Symptoms worsen, libido drops, and she all but gives up on herself as a sexual being.

One of the first things the average physician will do to treat a woman who shows up with PMS or difficult, irregular, painful or heavy periods—classic symptoms of estrogen dominance—is to prescribe birth control pills. Some birth control pills contain combinations of estrogens and synthetic progesterone (progestins), while others are progestin-only. Either kind of pill will make estrogen dominance worse. And the Pill further decreases libido by raising levels of sex hormone-binding globulin (SHBG) and lowering testosterone levels.

Many of the women I see in my practice have been on birth control pills for ten years or more. They don't realize that the Pill affects libido. Some women with estrogen dominance symptoms feel better on the Pill for a short time; at least their periods are less painful and heavy and they come on a regular schedule. Their other symptoms may also subside temporarily. But then, because the Pill makes the underlying problems worse, symptoms tend to re-emerge and worsen over time. When this happens, a woman can end up getting a hysterectomy she doesn't really need. Or, if a woman's symptoms show up primarily as a combination of agitation and depression or as big mood swings, she might end up being prescribed antidepressants—many of which cause a loss of libido.

The last two things most women in their 40s need is additional estrogen and progestins. The best way to reduce symptoms of estrogen dominance and restore libido is to use natural progesterone—a bioidentical version of the hormone made by the ovaries. If there are issues of stress, poor diet or thyroid problems, or if there are unresolved relationship issues, those need to be dealt with too. Progesterone is not a magical panacea, but it's a good place to begin.

Some women are reluctant to give up the Pill because it provides them with reliable contraception that doesn't involve surgery. I do my best to convince them that hormonal birth control isn't worth the cost to their health and their libidos.

If you aren't done having children or would like a reversible form of contraception for other reasons, I recommend a Paragard IUD (the kind *without* hormones) or barrier methods like condoms, diaphragms or cervical caps. For permanent birth control, consider a vasectomy for him or tubal blocking or ligation for yourself. Newer techniques for blocking the fallopian tubes can be done in a doctor's office.

A few research studies suggest that vasectomy may slightly increase a man's risk of prostate cancer or autoimmune disease. Some evidence also exists that tubal ligation may lead to changes in hormone levels, heavier/longer/more difficult periods, or early onset of menopause, also known as post-tubal ligation syndrome. Women who have a history of difficult periods seem to be at greater risk for this syndrome. Post-surgical complications are more common with tubal ligation than with vasectomy.

Overall, though, for each of these methods of contraception, there seems to be no consistent evidence that the risks of vasectomy or tubal ligation are significant enough to take them out of the running as valid, highly effective methods of birth control.

Testing and prescriptions for estrogen dominance

Symptoms can say a lot about whether a woman is estrogen dominant, but I always test estrogen, testosterone and progesterone levels before giving any hormones. When I suspect estrogen dominance, I also test thyroid hormones and adrenal hormones because these hormones interact with the hormones of libido in ways that influence the treatments I prescribe.

If a premenopausal woman proves estrogen dominant, bioidentical progesterone can help restore balance. Cortisol levels help me decide what type of progesterone to prescribe:

- Transdermal (applied to the skin) progesterone cream, which is available over-the-counter or from a compounding pharmacy, works well for raising progesterone levels just enough to achieve balance.

- If cortisol is high, I usually recommend oral progesterone (given in pill form). I also recommend oral progesterone for women who have difficulty sleeping because it acts as a mild sleep aid.

More particulars about dose, forms and schedules for using natural progesterone can be found in Chapter 4.

Reduce exposure to xenoestrogens

I also suggest that women who are estrogen dominant (and really, anyone else who wants to maintain healthy hormone balance and avoid carcinogens) reduce exposure to environmental estrogens (xenoestrogens) as much as possible by:

- Eating organic/pesticide-free fruits, vegetables, dairy products and eggs, and choosing free-range meats

- Avoiding meats, cheeses, oils and other fat-rich foods packaged in plastic containers; re-packaging foods packaged in plastic as soon as they get home from the store

- Avoid eating food from cans, which are lined with bisphenol A (BPA) containing plastic, as much as possible

- Using natural cleaning products that don't contain petrochemicals

- Finding alternatives to chemical pest control, including the pesticides used to prevent fleas in house pets

- Using cosmetics and body care products that don't contain unhealthy ingredients such as xenoestrogens, parabens and pthlatates (see the Environmental Working Group's continually updated list of safe products at **www.cosmeticsdatabase.com**)

- Using non-toxic, environmentally safe building products, paints and cleaners

- Using cast-iron cookware instead of cookware coated with Teflon

Nutritional supplements for estrogen dominance

I also recommend a few nutritional supplements for estrogen dominance.

Chasteberry is a traditional herbal remedy for PMS, and it can be especially helpful for women who get irritable around that time of the month. Although chasteberry originally got its name from its supposed libido-dampening effect (it's also called "monk's berry"), the use that has persisted over the centuries is as a fertility enhancer and hormone balancer.

Indole-3-carbinol is found in cruciferous vegetables like broccoli, cauliflower and cabbage. Research shows that it helps the body to more efficiently break down and get rid of excess estrogens. This likely explains why eating lots of cruciferous vegetables reduces risk of hormone-linked cancers like breast and prostate cancer.

Ground flaxseed also helps rid the body of extra estrogen. Eating plenty of fiber helps as well, by binding excess estrogen in the digestive tract and helping to move it out of the body more efficiently. This prevents the re-absorption of xenoestrogens through the wall of the large intestine. Substances found in flaxseed help the body switch out the stronger, more active forms of estrogen with milder *phytoestrogens* (plant forms of estrogen). Flaxseeds begin to go rancid immediately after the seeds are ground, so only use freshly ground seeds and never heat them. They can be ground in a coffee grinder.

B vitamins are important for detoxification—the process that breaks down toxins like xenoestrogens and flushes them out of the body—and so I also like to make sure that estrogen dominant patients are following the recommendations for B complex supplementation in Chapter 6. In some cases, I recommend a detoxification program to help flush as many xenoestrogens out of the body as possible.

When Relationship Issues are Part of the Problem (and They Almost Always Are)

There are women whose relationships are on track and whose libido issues are 100 percent physical, but they are the exception. The majority of women (and men) whose libidos go south in their 40s won't be able to bring their sex lives back to life without also taking a clear-eyed look at their relationship to the person with whom they want to be having sex.

I'm not a psychiatrist and don't claim to be qualified to help anyone sort through their marital problems. I am, however, a 40-something married woman whose libido went from lost to found, due in part to work done by my husband and myself on our relationship. The path that worked for us was Imago Relationship Therapy, which was developed by psychologist Harville Hendrix, Ph.D., and his wife and partner, Helen Lakelly Hunt, Ph.D.

There are many effective ways to do relationship work, and by endorsing one, I don't mean to dismiss any others—but many of my patients have found that Hendrix's work is simple, clear and very helpful. It's accessible even to those who don't wish to go to a therapist but who are willing to read Hendrix's books (they have written nine, including *Getting the Love You Want* and *Keeping the Love You Find*) with their partners and to put the books' advice into action in their relationships.

The word *Imago* is Latin for "image." Here, it describes a therapeutic model that helps to explain why couples are attracted to one another in the first place and why that attraction so often evolves into conflict as the first blush of romantic love wears off.

As we all know—whether we're parents ourselves or have just been raised by parents—almost all parents, even those who strive to be the best parents they can be, fall short in some way. At some point, the child feels afraid, lost, unloved or hurt by his or her parents. That's just the natural way of things. The emotional "map" created in the child by hurts both small and large is what Hendrix calls the Imago. It's carried into adulthood and affects the ways in which we relate to the world and to each other.

According to this model, we're drawn to partners who remind us of the people who raised us. We choose someone who fits into our emotional map—who loves us in a way that feels familiar because it recalls the love we got from our parents, complete with the flaws and difficulties that exist in every parent-child relationship. As adults, our Imago causes us to unconsciously seek out people who are most likely to bring those old difficulties back out into the light of day. Hendrix puts it this way: "We look for someone with the same deficits of care and attention that hurt us in the first place." When we do find that person, we feel strong, deep love in part because "our old brain is telling us that we've found someone with whom we can finally get our needs met."

Then, of course, the honeymoon ends, and this person we thought we could count on to fulfill our needs ends up refusing to do so. We feel betrayed—this couldn't possibly be the person with whom we were once so smitten. Couples often start to blame each other for the relationship's deterioration. As arguments and fights fail to resolve anything, dissatisfied partners become "ships passing in the night." They lose their sense of connection. No surprise then, when couples who are either in the arguing/ blaming stage or in the ships-passing-in-the-night stage start to have issues with lack of libido.

For an infant or small child who is incapable of caring for him or herself, not having the love of the parents is a life-or-death situation. We all developed fail-safe tactics for making sure we got the love we needed to survive. The emotional mind doesn't make the distinction between those childhood needs and the needs of adulthood. When we feel as though we are not getting the love we need, our emotional "brain" sends out the red alert. It *feels* like a life-or-death situation. Just understanding this can go a long way toward healing a relationship that has been broken down by fights, arguments, blaming and criticism.

In researching the communication styles of hundreds of couples, John Gottman, Ph.D., another psychologist, found that couples who fight are less likely to divorce than couples who have basically given up on fighting—who are tired and no longer trying to connect or get their needs met in their marriage. Imago therapy echoes this truth, seeing marital conflict not as a reason to separate, but as an opportunity. "The conflict isn't the problem, it's the answer," Hendrix writes. Conflict is a way *back* to intimacy with your partner. When you and your spouse are arguing over his having left his stinky socks in the middle of the bathroom floor, there's a much deeper issue at hand: the unmet needs of each partner. Until this "deeper emotional content" is explored and understood, Hendrix says, arguments will keep coming up, and partners might decide that they just can't get along or that the other person needs to change to make the relationship work.

Through Imago therapy, partners learn in depth about one another's emotional history. They learn that actually, this person they are trying to reason with is *not* insane—that his or her stance during disagreements makes perfect sense in the context of his or her past. In understanding this about the other person, each partner can move away from being defensive and critical and into a place of understanding.

Imago therapy gives simple guidelines about how to have conversations that create compassion and acceptance. This, in turn, strengthens love and mutual appreciation. Instead of reacting to each other with judgment, criticism, and attempts to get the other partner to change, partners begin to want to find ways to meet each other's unmet needs. Intimacy returns, and the way is paved for a renewed sexual connection.

Imago therapy sees committed relationships as an opportunity to bring people together in a context where each partner can repair lingering damage from early life, which then helps each partner become a happier, more fulfilled, more highly accomplished person. Your love for your partner and the life you have created together are strong motivations to stay and work things out. This person who seems to be bent on driving you crazy may actually be the ideal person to help you grow and change in positive ways.

More information about Imago therapy, workshops, and resources can be found at Hendrix's website, **www.harvillehendrix.com**.

Helping Him Get What He Wants

Women in their 40s often find themselves caught in a stressful juggling act because they're keeping so many balls in the air: raising children, working, caring for the home, dealing with finances… not to mention maintaining a relationship with a partner. It's no wonder that sex lives fall low on priority lists.

If your partner is pushing for more sex, let him know that one of the best female libido-enhancers around is the guy who helps with the housework, does his part with the kids, and otherwise takes on some of his partner's load. Try to talk through what he might do to help out more—and take care to do it in as non-confrontational a way as possible. Try to be positive and appreciative. For every task and responsibility he helps take off of your plate, he'll be rewarded with a partner who has more energy and desire to enjoy intimate time together.

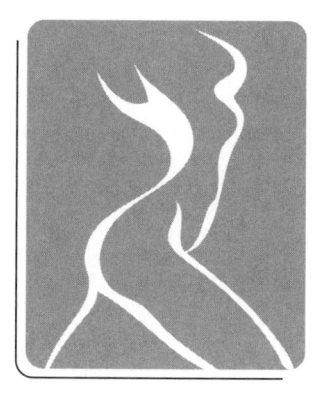

CHAPTER 13

The Fifties and Beyond – Menopause

When Marilyn came for her first office visit with me, she said, "You're my last hope—I feel as if I'm losing everything!" Her litany of complaints included no sex drive, vaginal dryness, hot flashes, night sweats, insomnia and "grouchiness." She had been on PremPro, and her doctor had taken her off it after evidence of thickening of the uterine lining, and was dropping hints that a hysterectomy might be the next step. Marilyn's eyes filled with tears as she said, "My husband is mad at me all the time because I don't want to have sex—it hurts! When my kids come home from college I yell at them about picking up after themselves, so they don't want to be around me. My OB/GYN wants me to take sleeping pills, but they make me fuzzy-headed so I can't function at work. If you can't help me I may end up unemployed, divorced and alone. My mother never had these problems; what's wrong with me?"

After reassuring Marilyn that, working as a team, we could do a lot to ease her symptoms, I also explained to her that her mother's menopause was likely far different from her own.

Not Your Mother's Menopause

If you're 50-something or older, chances are good that your father went off to work each day and your mother stayed home to take care of the kids. Your mother's retirement plan was probably that when you and your siblings were out of the house, and your father was retired, the two of them would live happily ever after, traveling and visiting with the grandkids. Your mother probably never mentioned menopause, and although she may have heard of estrogen, probably didn't take it unless you were from an upper middle class family. (If your mother did take estrogen-only HRT, there's a 60 percent chance she had to get a hysterectomy or got endometrial cancer.) Your mother's libido was probably low after menopause, and her expectation was that her sex life was over. Your father probably smoked cigarettes or cigars, had a few cocktails or beers before and after dinner, and had a significant gut created by eating lots of meat and potatoes, not to mention jello or cake for dessert every night; therefore he probably had a low libido and trouble getting and maintaining erections. So much for sex among 50-somethings in your parents' generation. They didn't expect a sex life after 50, didn't talk about it, and therefore didn't worry about it too much.

If you're a 50-something baby boomer, you and your partner have a dramatically different lifestyle and higher expectations. I say partner, because there's a 50 percent chance that you're divorced and a 25 percent chance that you're remarried, so if you're having sex there's a good chance it's with someone you're not married to. The other 25 percent of you may be interested in reviving your libido so that you can get back into the dating scene with some sexual confidence.

Having a sex life after 50 is, in some respects, a new frontier. As I pointed out above, today's cultural expectations are higher; couples want to keep having good sex into their golden years (and they can!). But today there are also, more than ever, deterrents to a good sex life after 50. The majority of women in the workplace have tired adrenals, which in turn depletes the sex hormones, so before we can even talk about better orgasms, we need to restore adrenal function. We are continuously exposed to estrogen-like substances (xenoestrogens) from plastics, pesticides, scented laundry soaps and air fresheners, nail polish, cosmetics, fiberboard, carpets and meat. This exposure is a setup for hormone imbalance in general and estrogen dominance in particular. Few conditions will make a woman feel less sexy than estrogen dominance, with its weight gain, puffiness, low thyroid, anxiety and irritability. We have more distractions than ever before, with cell phones, TV, Internet, email, Netflix and video games. If you're flopped on the couch after dinner, weary after a long day at work, what's going to be more appealing: sex with your husband of 20 years, or your favorite TV show and a bowl of ice cream? (Yet another reason why I recommend scheduling sex.)

I will be the first one to encourage you to have higher expectations than your parents did about sex after 50, but I'll also be the first one to tell you that your great new sex life won't be found in a pill, fad diet or magic exercise machine. Getting your sexy back is much more mundane than that, which is the good news and the bad news. It's the good news because anyone can do it, and the bad news because it involves those daily, routine decisions such as turning off the TV news to go for a walk; choosing a salad instead of fries at the restaurant, and insisting that your husband shave and take care of his ear and nose hair so that in your eyes, he can get his sexy back too.

Another essential part of creating a healthy sex life after 50 is figuring out what *you* really need, and asking for it. You have probably attended to the needs of others for decades, and this is a time to rediscover yourself. Christiane Northrup, M.D., shares wonderful insights about menopause in her books and TV specials. Part of her message is that women in midlife have an exciting opportunity to give birth to a new, vital and creative self. In *The Secret Pleasures of Menopause*, (Hay House 2008) she says, "Indulging in our passions is an important part of our midlife passage because it helps us connect at a deep emotional level with our newly emerging selves. Doing what we love and what brings us pleasure keeps our life force well-stoked… In fact, this feeling of being in love with life itself is absolutely vital if you want to have a passionate, fulfilling relationship with a partner…you can't give what you don't have."

Menopause Confusion

Confusion is the operative word for a woman in or approaching menopause these days. Although 40 percent of women move through the menopausal transition with minimal or moderate symptoms and distress, that leaves 60 percent who are coping with a grab bag of ever-changing symptoms and issues ranging from low libido, hot flashes and vaginal dryness to lack of confidence, weight gain and wrinkles. When, like Marilyn, they look for safe and effective solutions, they're met with conflicting advice from their girlfriends, doctors, the news media, drug company advertising, and a seemingly endless array of blogs and websites devoted to the 50-something woman.

Mainstream doctors are just as likely to be confused as their patients. They are bombarded with conflicting information from drug company reps, and if they keep up with medical journals, the research is often muddied by conflicts of interest, incomplete data and fuzzy conclusions. The 2002 Women's Health Initiative (WHI) research made it clear that women who use HRT, primarily PremPro, have a significantly increased risk of stroke, breast cancer, heart attack and gallbladder disease. Millions of women abruptly stopped using HRT after the WHI research came out and suffered for it.

Get Real and then Get Creative

Fifty-something women looking for their lost libido aren't simply dealing with low hormones; they're also experiencing the very real physical and emotional effects of aging, empty nests and a workplace that favors younger employees. Overall, women age more quickly than men; women start showing their age in the early 50s, while men who are in good physical condition can go until their late 50s or early 60s before they experience significant wrinkles, creaky joints, prostate problems and erectile dysfunction. Single men in their 50s and 60s are likely to be looking for women who are in their 40s and 50s—ten to 20 years younger. For single women looking for a sex partner, this inequity in aging and dating ages can lead to fad diets, Botox, tummy tucks and a bathroom cabinet full of anti-wrinkle creams.

I'm going to cover some of the symptoms of aging that can sap your sex drive, but I'd also like to make an argument for a certain amount of acceptance of the aging process. It's all very well to don a mumu, embrace your inner crone and celebrate menopausal zest, or at the other end of the spectrum spend tens of thousands of dollars on plastic surgery, Botox and personal trainers. The middle road is where most women end up. Regardless of whether you're dancing and chanting in a circle by firelight, or working out at the gym and heading to the beauty salon for hours every day, aging is inevitable. I don't care how many hormones you're taking, or how much freshly squeezed vegetable juice you guzzle, you are aging, you are wrinkling, your eyesight and hearing are going, your hair is turning white, and your joints are getting worn. So along with staying as healthy as possible, I recommend a good dose of reality therapy, or as sage Byron Katie says, learn to love reality, or learn to love what is. Minimize the regrets from the past and the fears of the future, and maximize what you have to work with. For some women that will mean new-found freedoms and creative explorations. For others the aging process will usher in a new era of discipline and taking care of the body. From the reality of wherever you are right now, you can add the hormones, the vitamins and the personal care regimens that appeal to you personally.

How Aging Can Sink Your Sex Life (and what you can do about it)

I'm not going to lie to you and pretend that if you exercise enough, eat all the right foods and have perfectly balanced hormones that the effects of aging won't still affect your sex life. Aging happens. The first task on the priority list for a 50-something woman is to get over it; ignore it when you can, and do your best with the rest. And that's not always easy; aging gracefully is an art. At some point during the 50s, regardless of genetics, lifestyle or plastic surgery, every woman looks in the mirror and realizes that the inevitable is very much in progress. So, my first prescription for libido restoration for menopausal women is acceptance.

All of the issues mentioned below are covered in more detail in other chapters, but it's important to be aware that any of these issues, alone or together, can contribute to a low libido.

Even if you've managed to keep your weight low through the 40s, your body is responding to the inexorable call of gravity. That tight butt is more like a jello butt, those thighs have telltale signs of cottage cheese, the upper arm flesh jiggles when you wave (and keeps jiggling), and of course sags and wrinkles are appearing on your face. Unless you have kept your hands under the protection of white gloves for a lifetime, you're getting age spots on the back of your hands. And let's not forget varicose veins, bags under the eyes, saggy eyelids and buckling teeth. All this change in the space of a few years can be intimidating and sap self-confidence; not a good recipe for a healthy libido. This is why I recommend laying the foundation for a great sex life after 50 by first accepting what is, and then using my guidelines to optimize your health and libido.

A lack of self-esteem will deflate your sexy a lot faster than vaginal dryness, which can be remedied with hormone replacement and lubricants. What's going to be most sexy to the man in your life is your confidence, enthusiasm, and most of all your full attention and participation.

Weight

The first symptom of aging that most women notice is the tendency to gain weight and the redistribution of weight. This begins as early as the mid-30s, but by menopause it's hard to ignore. Some weight gain is natural and normal, but excessive weight gain will sap energy and decrease libido due to poor blood flow. When blood can't get to the sexual organs, physical arousal cannot occur, even when the brain is willing.

I strongly recommend the nutrition and exercise solutions covered in other chapters and a "just do it" attitude toward taking the necessary steps to maintain a healthy weight after menopause. The rewards are far greater than the sacrifices.

Sight

Most women need reading glasses by the time they reach menopause. It's worth spending the time and money to find glasses that are stylish and make you feel sexy. Dry eyes are a common symptom of estrogen deficiency and can cause bloodshot eyes and chronic eye irritation. Chronic eye irritation doesn't look or feel good. Wearing sunglasses, managing allergies and hormone balance can all help.

Creaky joints

The more exercise you've done in your life, the earlier you'll probably notice that your joints don't work as well as they used to. This doesn't seem fair, but it's a simple matter of wear and tear. Well-used joints wear out faster. Sore hips can be a real libido buster—it's not sexy for you or him if you're grunting with pain when you spread your legs. By far the best remedy for creaky joints is movement. It's important to do gentle stretching when you get up in the morning and to move and stretch throughout the day. Maintaining good muscle tone will help the muscles, tendons and ligaments support the joints.

Dry va-jay-jay

As coined by Oprah, dry va-jay-jay, or a dry vagina is one of the hallmark symptoms of aging, menopause and estrogen deficiency, and is easily remedied with estrogen. If needed, vaginal estrogens and testosterone can very effectively restore the vagina to its pre-menopausal health. *For details see chapters 3 and 4.*

Sagging organs

Gravity doesn't just take its toll on the skin, it's also at work on our organs, stretching out the tendons, ligaments and other types of tissue that hold our organs in place. Many women suffer from a degree of prolapse, or sagging of the uterus or bladder that can interfere with sex. Your doctor may recommend surgery to shore up the organs, but unless absolutely necessary this is not an ideal solution because it can create scar tissue and adhesions that can cause more discomfort than the prolapse. BHRT and Kegel exercises combined with weight loss and fitness can dramatically reverse prolapse, and I have numerous patients who have avoided surgery.

Hot flashes and night sweats

No woman who feels like it's 120 degrees Fahrenheit in the room and who is soaking the sheets with sweat is going to feel sexy, but hormone balancing is the ultimate hot flash and night sweats solution. For women who prefer not to use hormones, herbal remedies such as red clover extract and black cohosh can be helpful. Otherwise, if you wait it out for a year or two, both the hot flashes and the night sweats will gradually go away.

Moodiness

Irritability, weepiness, depression, anxiety—none of these emotional states are likely to enhance sexual arousal in you or your mate. Putting aside the possibility that you may need some counseling, hormone balance can work wonders for most kinds of mood instability. Women who are suffering from moodiness usually need more than the basic duo of estrogen and progesterone—an adrenal makeover is also in order. For women who wish to avoid hormones, fish oil can act as a wonderful mood stabilizer.

Insomnia

It's certainly not sexy when a woman falls asleep during foreplay because she's been tossing and turning, hot flashing and sweating all night. Sleep deprivation makes all of the menopausal symptoms worse, but for most women, some simple lifestyle changes and hormone balancing will banish night sweats and bring back restful sleep. In fact, progesterone alone will help most women sleep soundly through the night. Also, be aware that excess estrogen or testosterone can cause insomnia. Herbal sleep remedies often work well to support good sleep.

Disappearing parts

When hormone levels drop, a woman's sexual parts tend to shrink, with the exception of the inner labia, which tend to stretch. A low-hormone vagina can shrink so much that a finger can't even be inserted, making insertion of an erect penis out of the question. A clitoris deprived of testosterone can virtually disappear and become insensitive, or even hypersensitive in a bad way (feeling like any stimulation feels like sandpaper rubbing on the clitoris) rendering a major pleasure center out of commission. A G-spot deprived of estrogen and testosterone can become unresponsive to stimulation. The perineum, which is the skin between the vagina and anus, is wider in premenopausal woman than in men, but in a menopausal women with low hormones, it can become very narrow and prone to irritation during sex. This narrowing can contribute to urinary tract infections. When hormone levels are restored, these important zones of sexuality plump up again, stretch out again, and become more sensitive and responsive.

Bioidentical Hormone Confusion

Trying to find a doctor to help with bioidentical hormone balancing can be challenging because there is so much conflicting information on the subject. The information provided in this book will provide you with a good foundation for making a good choice. Just remember: use bioidentical hormones only when needed and in doses that mimic what your body would naturally make.

Many women come to see me after taking bioidentical hormones and having a bad experience almost always caused by what I call mega-dosing. Mega-dosing occurs because improperly trained doctors don't understand how different types of hormone applications behave differently in the body. They prescribe a progesterone and estrogen cream, for example, measure hormone levels with a serum blood test, and find that hormone levels have not gone up, so they increase the dose. Unfortunately it takes an elephant-sized dose of hormones to get transdermal (through the skin) hormones to show up in a serum blood test. What these doctors don't realize is that transdermal hormones are not found in the serum part of the blood, so unless mega-doses are used, they will never show up on their test! Mega-dose hormones, bioidentical or otherwise, can and do cause serious health problems, most often rapid weight gain, hair loss, fatigue, and insomnia. Excess estrogen can cause extreme anxiety and irritability. Of greater concern is that mega-doses of hormones can lead to an increase in risk of uterine cancers.

You can refer back to Chapter 4 for recommendations on how to test hormone levels.

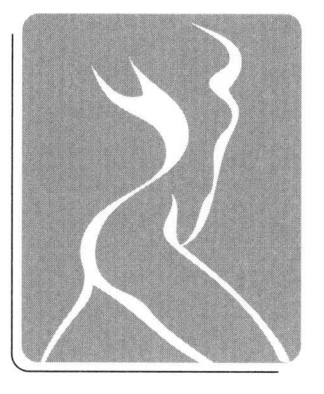

CHAPTER 14

Where Did it Go?
The Libido Quiz

A s you probably realize by now, there are plenty of places that a libido can disappear into, from piles of dirty laundry and hormone imbalances, to bedroom boredom and medications.

If it's not clear by now what's sinking your sex life, this quiz can help you zero in on specific areas that can be addressed.

Each question is given a rating of 1 to 5, with 1 being "not true" and 5 being "very true." Circle the number that best describes you. When you've answered all of the questions with a rating number, add the numbers within each group and write down the total. The groups with the *lowest* totals are where you might want to begin your libido reboot.

Go to the end of the chapter to find solutions for your group(s).

Group 1

	Not True	↔		Very True
I'm happy with my sexual partner.	1 2	3	4	5
I'm sexually attracted to my partner.	1 2	3	4	5
My partner and I communicate well.	1 2	3	4	5
My partner knows how to meet my sexual needs.	1 2	3	4	5
My partner and I have a mutually fulfilling sexual relationship.	1 2	3	4	5

TOTAL: _____

Group 2

	Not True	↔		Very True
My partner and I equally divide household, family and financial responsibilities.	1 2	3	4	5
I feel supported and appreciated by my partner.	1 2	3	4	5
I'm getting enough sleep and rest.	1 2	3	4	5
I take time every day for meditation/contemplation.	1 2	3	4	5
I'm managing the stress in my life.	1 2	3	4	5

TOTAL: _____

Group 3

	Not True	↔		Very True
I feel good about my body.	1 2	3	4	5
I feel good about my sexuality.	1 2	3	4	5
I'm confident in my sexuality.	1 2	3	4	5
I know what turns me on and how to communicate that.	1 2	3	4	5
I'm a good sexual partner.	1 2	3	4	5

TOTAL: _____

Group 4

	Not True	↔		Very True
I eat healthy foods.	1 2 3 4 5			
I rarely eat fast foods.	1 2 3 4 5			
I eat organic whenever possible.	1 2 3 4 5			
Sugar and refined carbs are an occasional treat.	1 2 3 4 5			
I eat plenty of whole grains and veggies.	1 2 3 4 5			

TOTAL: _____

Group 5

	Not True	↔		Very True
I exercise daily.	1 2 3 4 5			
I exercise enough to maintain a healthy weight.	1 2 3 4 5			
My exercise routine is enjoyable.	1 2 3 4 5			
I consider myself physically fit.	1 2 3 4 5			
I make daily exercise a priority.	1 2 3 4 5			

TOTAL: _____

Group 6 (Premenopausal)

	Not True	↔		Very True
My periods are regular.	1 2 3 4 5			
I don't have PMS.	1 2 3 4 5			
I don't have polycystic ovary syndrome (PCOS).	1 2 3 4 5			
I regularly feel sexually aroused.	1 2 3 4 5			
My moods are reasonably stable.	1 2 3 4 5			

TOTAL: _____

Group 7

	Not True	↔		Very True	
I don't have water weight (edema, bloating).	1	2	3	4	5
I'm able to manage moods and emotions.	1	2	3	4	5
I'm able to fall asleep and stay asleep.	1	2	3	4	5
I don't have a lot of excess weight around my hips and thighs.	1	2	3	4	5
My memory is good and thinking is clear.	1	2	3	4	5

TOTAL: _____

Group 8 (Menopausal)

	Not True	↔		Very True	
Intercourse is pain-free.	1	2	3	4	5
My vagina is well-lubricated during sex.	1	2	3	4	5
I have few or manageable hot flashes.	1	2	3	4	5
I have little or no night sweats.	1	2	3	4	5
I am able to become sexually aroused (with or without my partner).	1	2	3	4	5

TOTAL: _____

Low Sex Drive Solutions

Group 1 – Relationship Repair

Invest in quality time with your partner and if necessary get some couples counseling.

Review chapters 10 and 12.

Group 2 – Self Support

Time to take better care of yourself.

Review chapters 8 and 9.

Group 3 – Sexual Self-Confidence

When lifestyle issues such as diet, exercise and hormone balance are addressed, sexual self confidence often returns.

Review chapters 4, 8 and 9.

Group 4 – Healthy Eating

This is one of the foundations of a healthy lifestyle, and better energy.

Review chapter 9.

Group 5 – Exercise

Another foundation of a healthy lifestyle and better energy—just do it—no excuses!

Review the Pro-Libido Workout Plan in chapter 9.

Group 6 – Premenopausal Hormone Fluctuations

The hormonal ups and downs of the 40s can sink your sex life. Healthy lifestyle and a little bit of progesterone may help.

Review chapter 12.

Group 7 – Estrogen Dominance

An imbalance between progesterone and estrogen can wreak hormone havoc. Time to get your hormone levels tested.

Review chapters 4, 5 and 12.

Group 8 – Estrogen Deficiency

Low estrogen can contribute to vaginal dryness and shrinking, as well as hot flashes and night sweats. It may be time for some supplemental estrogen and progesterone.

Review chapter 12 or 13.

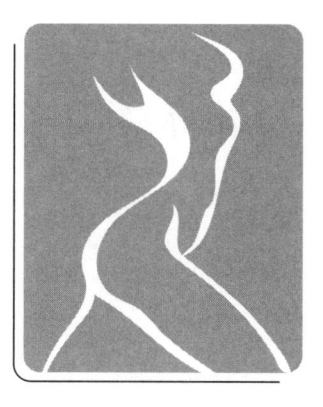

CHAPTER 15

What If It's Him, Not Me?

When I first began to shift my practice from obstetrics and gynecology to hormone balancing, many of my female patients would say, "You've helped me so much. What can you do for my husband?"

I was a little nervous about working with male patients, not having done so since medical school. But when I began to expand my knowledge to include men in my practice, I found that while balancing hormones in women can be a juggling act, doing so with men is a snap! Attaining balance involves just one hormone in many cases. Of course, the other aspects of restoring libido—including nutrition, exercise, mindfulness and communication—apply just as much for men as they do for women. But dealing with the hormonal aspect is far simpler in men than in women.

In this chapter, you'll learn what can send a man's libido south and how he can restore it. When both partners have a balanced libido, the sparks can really fly.

Libido Problems in Men: An Overview

A drop in libido is rarer for men than for women, but an estimated 16 percent of men do experience low libido. They may try to avoid sex altogether even if their partners are raring to go. Sometimes libido sinks because of physical problems like erectile dysfunction (ED). Sometimes, as is the case with women, sex drive drops because of relationship problems, fatigue, stress, anxiety or physical illness. Low testosterone almost always plays a role.

Sexual dysfunction affects about 30 percent of men at one time or another. For some, the problems are strictly physical. Erectile dysfunction (ED) affects 12 percent of men under age 40, 18 percent of men aged 50 to 59, and 25 to 30 percent of men over 60. One in three men experiences premature ejaculation at least some of the time. Performance anxiety, which (not surprisingly) often goes along with premature ejaculation or ED, affects about one in every five men.

A man's identity and masculinity tend to be tied into his sexuality, and when this part of himself is not up to par, the rest of his life is strongly impacted. A survey of men and women who had experienced loss of libido found that while 46 percent of the women felt happy with their lives in general despite their sexual difficulties, only 23 percent of the men had the same general contentment with their lives when their sex lives weren't satisfactory.

The causes of male sexual dysfunction in midlife can be hormonal, psychological or social. They can be caused by health problems like cardiovascular disease, prostate disease or diabetes. Let's look at the issues your partner might be facing and how they can be addressed.

Erectile Dysfunction (ED)

When a man doesn't get erections hard enough or long-lasting enough for satisfying sex, the diagnosis is ED. He may only be able to stay hard for a little while or he may not get hard at all.

The relationship between libido and arousal is complex in men, but not quite as complex as it is in women. Generally, if a man doesn't want sex, he doesn't get an erection, but if he can't get an erection, he *still* might want sex! (Remember that women can become aroused physically and still have no libido.) While a woman's lack of arousal doesn't necessarily show, when a man doesn't get hard, a sexual encounter might grind to a halt on an unpleasant note. That's a lot of pressure! And for a man who'd rather be in denial about ED or who feels embarrassment about it, not attempting to have sex is one way to avoid facing the problem.

In past decades, ED wasn't something a man was comfortable talking about, even with a physician. This has changed—especially since the introduction of highly effective drugs to treat ED. But going to a doctor to get a prescription for Viagra, Cialis or Levitra shouldn't be the end of the story for a man with ED. Some underlying issues believed to cause or contribute to ED can be addressed with the diet and lifestyle shifts described in other chapters of this book. For some men, hormone replacement may be an important part of restoring better erectile function.

Physical causes of ED

Cardiovascular disease. The blood vessels that bring blood into the penis to create an erection can narrow because of fatty deposits or hardening of the arteries.

Obesity. Obesity and overweight affect cardiovascular health in ways that can hamper erectile function. Obesity alters hormone balance, raising estrogen levels and lowering testosterone levels—which doesn't promote good erectile function.

Diabetes. Both type 1 (insulin-dependent) and type 2 (adult-onset) diabetes affect the health of nerves and blood vessels throughout the body. Thirty to 50 percent of diabetic men have ED. Good diabetes control is key for maintaining healthy erectile function.

Hormone imbalance. Testosterone naturally declines in men as they age. Low testosterone affects both erectile function and libido, and testosterone replacement can be a big help. This topic is covered in more depth later in this chapter.

Prescription medications. Antidepressants, blood pressure medicines, antihistamines, tranquilizers, cholesterol-lowering drugs and the ulcer drug Tagamet (cimetidine) can all affect erectile function. So can the drug finasteride, which is used to treat prostate enlargement (in pill form) or hair loss (in topical or pill form). Drugs used to treat advanced prostate cancer have hormone-blocking effects that are almost certain to suppress libido and erectile function. Shifts in lifestyle and diet can help minimize the need for medications. When drugs are necessary, men can work with their doctors to find alternatives that don't impact erectile function or libido.

Stress. High stress can cause erectile dysfunction. Doing mindfulness practice, exercise, yoga, or other stress-relieving activities described in Chapter 8 will promote better sexual function and sensation for both of you—and it can bring you closer.

Prostate enlargement. In this common condition, a man's prostate swells and partly closes off the urethra so that urine doesn't flow efficiently from the bladder. It's also known as BPH (benign prostatic hypertrophy). Medications help get urine flowing again, but men with BPH are more likely to have erectile dysfunction, and the alpha-blocker medicines used to treat it can make the problem worse. So can alpha-reductase inhibitors like Proscar (finasteride) and Avodart (dutasteride).

Many men have success treating BPH with the herbs saw palmetto and pygeum, which may also have dampening effects on libido, but less so than the drugs.

Psychological factors. According to the Mayo Clinic, anxiety, depression, low self-esteem and fear of sexual inadequacy are implicated in 10 to 20 percent of cases of ED. Even when there is a physical cause for ED, that cause can be compounded if a man becomes stressed or anxious around the problem.

Smoking and alcohol or drug abuse. Addiction to alcohol, nicotine or other drugs will affect erectile function and libido. The obvious solution is to get help and kick the addiction.

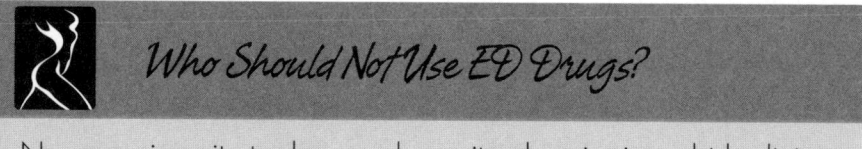

Who Should Not Use ED Drugs?

No one using nitrate drugs such as nitroglycerin, isosorbide dinitrate or isosorbide mononitrate should take any form of ED drug (Viagra, Cialis or Levitra).

ED drugs are almost always unsafe for men with history of stroke, blood clots, hypertension, low blood pressure, congestive heart failure, angina (heart pains), heart attack or heart rhythm problems. Any man who has had a heart attack or stroke within the past six months, or who has any medical condition that makes sexual activity dangerous (unstable angina, very high or very low blood pressure, liver disease) should not use Cialis.

Men with bleeding disorders, liver or kidney diseases, disorders of blood cells, stomach ulcers or inherited eye diseases should not use ED drugs.

Men who take alpha-blockers — which are prescribed to treat high blood pressure, prostate conditions and certain circulatory problems — need to use caution with ED medications. Cardura (doxazosin), Minipress (prazosin), Hytrin (terazosin), Flomax (tamsulosin) and Uroxatral (alfuzosin) are all alpha-blockers. Levitra should not be used at all with any alpha-blocker; Cialis is safe with only one kind of alpha-blocker (tamsulosin, brand name Flomax); Viagra can be used in the 25-mg dose with alpha-blockers, but if 50 or 100 mg are used, men are advised to wait at least four hours after taking their alpha-blocker.

Other causes of ED

Neurological disorders or spinal injury. Any health problem that damages nerves can affect erectile function. Multiple sclerosis, Parkinson's disease and spinal injury are examples.

Chronic liver or kidney disease. Not only can these conditions cause ED—they also preclude the use of ED drugs.

Prostate disease surgery. Surgical treatments for prostate disease can permanently damage nerves that are necessary for healthy erectile function.

For men with these conditions who can't use Viagra or related medicines (see the Sidebar for more on this), other avenues are available, including vacuum pumps, injectable medications and penile implants. None of these are as draconian as they sound. They are all useful ED treatments.

If ED can't be effectively treated medically, this is where the toys and novel approaches described in Chapter 10 come in handy—and where thinking outside the box about what sex is really about can be invaluable. An erect penis isn't a prerequisite for a loving, pleasurable sexual encounter!

Premature Ejaculation

During sexual intercourse, the normal span of time between vaginal penetration and ejaculation is between two and ten minutes. An estimated one in three men ejaculates prematurely at least some of the time—that is, within a minute after penetration, or sooner than he and/or his partner would like. When this happens often enough to create distress or leave either partner dissatisfied, the man might just decide he'd rather avoid sex because he thinks it's something he can't fix. The good news is that men with this problem can almost always fix it without medications of any kind.

When a man is stressed, is nervous or has performance anxiety, he's more likely to be unable to delay ejaculation. Anxiety over ED can create a pattern in which the man tries to ejaculate quickly, before he gets soft—a habit that becomes difficult to break. Unresolved relationship issues can cause premature ejaculation as well. If a man has not had problems with premature ejaculation before, the causes are probably primarily psychological.

Hormone imbalances, an abnormal ejaculatory reflex, thyroid disease, prostate or urethra inflammation (prostatitis/urethritis) or heredity can also play a role. Some psychiatric medications can cause premature ejaculation.

The best way to treat premature ejaculation is with sexual techniques that gradually train the man to delay ejaculation, without pharmaceutical help. After a period of doing these techniques alone, he'll develop control and a relaxed, mindful state that he can then bring to you during sex. And by the way, a man doesn't have to have premature ejaculation issues to benefit from this exercise—it can help any man to have more intense orgasms and have more control.

This next part is for men to read themselves, or it can be read aloud by their loving partners.

For men: Start/stop technique to delay ejaculation

The *start/stop technique* works like this:

1. Notice, the next time you masturbate or have sex, the tickling sensation that precedes ejaculation. Also notice the sensations that come before you reach the "point of no return." Don't use lubricants yet; those will be used later on, once you've gained more control.

2. Once you've taken the time to be mindful of those sensations, take some time on three different occasions to masturbate in a way that resembles intercourse—by stroking up and down on the penis. Keep paying close attention to the way it feels in the genitals and pelvis. Don't actively try *not* to ejaculate; simply become very familiar with the pre-tingle and the tingle that come right before ejaculation.

3. Then, begin with the start/stop exercise. Masturbate to the point of being aroused, then stop for 15 or more seconds and breathe deeply. Try to decrease the level of excitement in your genitals. Imagine that energy spreading out and around your whole body, from head to toe. Don't use fantasy here; your goal is to tune in as completely as possible to body sensations.

4. Begin masturbating again. Get aroused but stop short of that tickling/tingling phase that comes right before orgasm. Doing Kegel exercises can help maintain control when you get close to the edge. Your erection may come and go during a session, and that's fine. Get yourself right to the edge at least three times, then let yourself ejaculate. Continue breathing deeply and being mindful of your whole body as you do the exercise.

5. Keep doing this exercise every day if possible. Build up with the goal of getting close to orgasm six times before ejaculating.

6. Then, add a lubricant to make it feel more like the real thing. Go back to three start/stop cycles and build back up to six. This is where you can start to bring your partner in to support, witness and help—and eventually, to enjoy your new ability to last longer!

If a man sees a doctor for help with premature ejaculation, he may end up with a prescription for an antidepressant drug such as Zoloft, Paxil or Prozac. These drugs usually help to delay ejaculation, but they carry a high risk of reducing libido—not a great tradeoff! Another antidepressant called Anafranil (clomipramine) is sometimes prescribed to delay ejaculation. Condoms lined with anesthetic creams or topically applied anesthetic creams are another pharmaceutical tactic. The downside of these creams is the same thing that makes them delay ejaculation: reduced sensitivity. And sometimes, the female partner ends up having a reduction in sensitivity because traces of the medication end up in her vagina.

Delayed Ejaculation

Rarely, a man's ejaculatory problem may be the opposite of premature—he may not be able to ejaculate at all, or ejaculation may be delayed for more than a half hour during active intercourse. In some cases of delayed ejaculation, the man may only be able to ejaculate while masturbating alone, but not with a partner.

To a woman who enjoys sex and has a strong libido, delayed ejaculation might not sound like such a bad thing. But for couples who are trying to find a healthy, pleasurable middle ground, this situation can put unwelcome pressure on both partners. A woman who knows that any sexual encounter with her partner is going to last at least 30 minutes may not want to go there at all. A man who knows that he might not achieve orgasm or have to work very hard to get there might also decide it's not worth the effort to be sexual.

Delayed ejaculation can be caused by psychological factors (anxiety, overly strict religious background, lack of attraction, relationship issues or sexual trauma), physical problems (nerve damage, stroke, prostate disease, high blood pressure) or medications (SSRI antidepressants, anti-psychotics, blood pressure drugs, alcohol, opiate pain drugs, recreational drugs). If medications and physical problems don't turn out to be the cause, sex therapy is the best route. Psychological or couples counseling might be helpful, too. In most cases, delayed ejaculation can be successfully treated.

Andropause, Libido and Performance

Men don't go through the kind of abrupt hormonal shifts that women experience in their 40s and 50s. But their levels of testosterone do decline gradually, at the rate of about one to two percent per year. This change can eventually lead to a situation known as *andropause*, where testosterone activity drops far enough to affect his sex drive and erectile function.

When the following symptoms start to crop up for a man, low testosterone is a likely cause:

- low energy, fatigue
- reduced muscle mass
- fat gain that doesn't respond to exercise and dietary changes
- drop in libido
- erection problems
- sleeplessness
- gain in fat mass that isn't lost as easily as it once was

Andropause can make a guy feel like a grumpy old man. Stamina and competitive "edge" may fall, followed by self-esteem and confidence. The man may feel as though something's missing from his life, and in an effort to reclaim the energy and passion of his high-testosterone youth, he might go through the stereotypical midlife crisis—trying to assume the outward trappings of a younger man. For others, andropause brings depression and sadness. He may close himself off, leaving loved ones without much of a clue as to what's wrong or how to help. A man who is experiencing this but doesn't know about andropause will usually just figure that he's aging, and that this is what it's like—that there's nothing to be done about it.

Just as the mood swings and health issues of menopause can interfere with intimacy and libido, so too can the emotions, physical symptoms and behaviors that crop up around andropause. There's some evidence that men who are entering andropause today started out with lower testosterone levels than their fathers did—making for a lower threshold for andropausal symptoms to set in.

The Low-Testosterone Generation?

Men's testosterone levels are lower, on average, than their fathers' levels were at the same age. This is probably due to having been virtually bathed in estrogen-mimicking chemicals from before birth. Males' testosterone levels are influenced by this extra estrogenic burden. Men are also heavier overall than they were a generation ago; more fat means higher estrogen and lower levels of testosterone. Rising use of multiple prescription drugs has also been blamed for contributing to the overall drop in testosterone levels in modern men. Fortunately, bioidentical testosterone replacement is proving to be a safe, effective way to bring testosterone up to ideal levels in men whose health and well-being are affected by andropausal symptoms.

For a man whose testosterone levels are low, giving enough bioidentical hormone to get him into the optimal range can be truly transformative. In my practice, men who get appropriate testosterone replacement are amazed at how much better they feel and function.

When testosterone is low, replacement has many benefits

Testosterone promotes cardiovascular health, brain health, energy, libido and muscular strength. In aging men, it protects against heart disease, Alzheimer's disease and osteoporosis. When levels fall too low, men lose feelings of vitality, strength and youthfulness—and they may even lose years of life. One large study from the University of California in San Diego found that healthy men whose testosterone levels were low had a 33 percent greater risk of death in the next two decades than men whose testosterone was in the higher ranges.

The heart has more testosterone receptors than any other organ, which suggests that this hormone is important for keeping it healthy. There's a virtual mountain of evidence in favor of adequate testosterone levels helping to prevent heart attacks in men. Higher testosterone is linked with lower insulin levels, more healthy body weight, and healthier cholesterol and blood fat levels.

One fascinating study of rats found that when male rats were castrated, they began to develop cardiovascular disease; but when they were given supplemental testosterone, the disease actually began to reverse itself. Testosterone has direct effects on heart function and on the ability of blood vessels to work their best. Studies show that an infusion of testosterone, given to a man having a heart attack, improves his chances of recovering.

When testosterone dips too low, a man can begin to feel depressed. Research shows a strong association between depression, andropausal symptoms and low testosterone. Just as is the case with women, this symptom has nothing to do with a deficiency of Zoloft, or of any other antidepressant medication! Low testosterone should be high on the list of possible causes when a man who's entering or well into midlife becomes depressed or has other significant changes in mood. Some research points to a link between higher risk of dementia in older age and lower testosterone levels.

Defining low testosterone is trickier than you might think

Chad was a 45-year-old attorney who had lost energy, stamina and libido over the course of a few months. He had seen a magazine article that described the symptoms of low testosterone and had gone to his usual doctor for testing. "The results were normal," he told me when he came to see me with his wife Elizabeth. "So it has to be something else, right?" I explained to Chad that no, a "normal" result on a standard testosterone test didn't rule out a role for his testosterone levels in his symptoms.

There are two good reasons why standard tests for testosterone don't accurately reflect whether a man will benefit from bioidentical HRT:

1. To come up with "normal" levels of testosterone, testing labs like Quest Diagnostics measure testosterone levels in 10,000 or so men, all of whom are healthy and say that they feel fine. They average these levels out and come up with a range, which they then call "normal." Despite the fact that testosterone levels fall naturally with age, there's no adjustment of normal levels across a man's lifespan to reflect those changes. "Normal" testosterone, according to the standard tests used by most doctors, can be anything from 250 nanograms per deciliter (ng/dl) to 1100 ng/dl! So a man who's 40 can show up with a testosterone of 350 ng/dl and be told that this is within normal ranges. It is, but this is like telling a 40-year-old with the testosterone levels of a 70-year-old that he's within normal range. If he has andropausal symptoms too, I'd say his testosterone is low and that he might want to

consider replacement. The optimal range of total testosterone for a man is more like 800 ng/dl to 1100 ng/dl, which is the optimal level of testosterone for a man in his mid-20s. The goal here is to replace the testosterone to the higher part of the range or what doctors in my field refer to as the optimal range

2. Most doctors measure total testosterone only, instead of measuring free testosterone (the testosterone not tightly bound to sex hormone binding globulin or SHBG). Some testosterone is loosely bound to albumin, another protein found in the blood, and is easily accessed by the body when needed. Together, free and albumin-bound testosterone are considered *bioavailable.* Bound testosterone is biologically inactive. Any testosterone test that does not measure both free and bound portions won't give an accurate picture of testosterone activity in the body. A man can have high total testosterone with high levels of bound testosterone, which makes him functionally low. Or a man can have low total testosterone with low levels of bound testosterone, and replacement might not be needed. Optimal range for bioavailable testosterone is between 350 ng/dL and 575 ng/dL.

Testosterone replacement: Guidelines, precautions and benefits

When a man has classic andropausal symptoms and his testosterone levels could use some adjustment, a trial of testosterone replacement is the next step. A few important factors we consider:

Prostate cancer risk

In most medical practices, men with any history of prostate cancer within the last five years are advised not to use testosterone replacement, as it's theorized that it could help accelerate established cancer. In past years, there was some concern about testosterone replacement as a potential cause of prostate cancer. Those concerns have almost completely been laid to rest, and some doctors are finding that testosterone replacement reduces the risk of prostate cancer.

No association has been found between high-normal (optimal) testosterone levels and the diagnosis of prostate cancer. In fact, there's some evidence to the contrary—that higher testosterone may actually be protective against prostate cancer. In some long-term studies, men with the lowest testosterone have been found to have the highest prostate cancer risk and the most aggressive cancers. Higher levels of estrogens seem to pose greater risk of prostate cancer than high testosterone.

In men who have small, undiagnosed prostate cancers, there is some possibility that testosterone replacement might accelerate their growth. This is why men who are considering testosterone therapy are advised to have digital rectal exam (DRE) and prostate-specific antigen (PSA) tests first. We monitor PSA after starting testosterone therapy: at three months we do another test, and then every six months thereafter.

Benign prostate hypertrophy (BPH)

Men with BPH—prostate enlargement—sometimes experience worse symptoms when they use testosterone. Most have improvements, including less urinary hesitancy and less dribbling. When a man has worsening prostate problems after starting testosterone supplementation, it's an indication that he is converting more of that hormone into another form, *dihydrotestosterone* (DHT), which stimulates prostate growth. He may need small doses of medication to reduce the activity of an enzyme called 5-alpha-reductase, which transforms testosterone into DHT. High DHT is also implicated in male pattern baldness. A low dose of a 5-alpha-reductase inhibitor (Proscar, Avodart) may be helpful for men who convert a lot of testosterone to DHT. (These drugs can reduce libido unless the doses are properly controlled by checking levels.) Saw palmetto is a natural 5-alpha reductase inhibitor and can sometimes be used to slow the conversion of testosterone to DHT.

Transformation of testosterone to estrogens

Some men's bodies more readily transform testosterone into estrogens through a process called *aromatization*. Remember, estrogen is a *female* hormone. Because aromatization happens largely in fat cells, men who are obese or overweight are more likely to aromatize more testosterone and raise their estrogen levels too high. Men of normal weight can have this issue as well.

Giving testosterone to men who aromatize a lot of it to estrogen will cause estrogen levels to rise—which will either fail to improve andropausal symptoms and lack of libido or make them worse. Men whose estrogen levels rise too much relative to testosterone are also at risk for gynecomastia (growth of breasts), tenderness in the breast area and prostate cancer, and there may also be a negative impact on heart health when estrogen is too high.

Estrogen is good for men in the right balance with other hormones. It's important for bone and brain health as they age. Before I give testosterone replacement I test estrogen levels, and if they are high, I prescribe a small dose of a medication called an aromatase inhibitor such as Arimidex (anastrozole) along with the testosterone. I'm careful to do follow-up checks of estrogen and testosterone levels to make sure that aromatization isn't preventing the replacement hormone from doing its job.

Stress and cortisol

Encourage your partner to participate with you in your own stress-reducing strategies. Stress strongly affects the rate of decline of testosterone as well as its ability to bind to receptors. A man who is not taking steps to cope with work, relationship and other life stresses will have a much harder time balancing his hormones and improving his sex life.

High stress leads to high cortisol levels—which, eventually, can lead to adrenal fatigue, where cortisol levels fall too low. Tiredness, insomnia, new allergies or chemical sensitivities, reduced tolerance for stress and lower resistance to infection all suggest adrenal fatigue.

Men whose adrenals are exhausted may benefit from supplemental DHEA (dehydroepiandrosterone), the "parent hormone" from which estrogens, testosterone and cortisol are made. Although DHEA is available over-the-counter, I don't recommend using it without a doctor's guidance. Hormone levels need to be monitored while using DHEA to ensure that it's being used to make the hormones we want more of.

Thyroid health

Thyroid hormone levels are often low in andropausal men, and I test for this too, in order to ensure that we get the complete picture of thyroid hormone production and interconversion. Giving testosterone alone to a man whose thyroid hormones are out of balance won't solve his issues. He may need thyroid replacement too.

Fertility

Giving testosterone replacement has the paradoxical effect of reducing sperm count and causing testicular shrinkage (about 20 percent of total volume). Because the body is getting supplemental testosterone, it gets the message that testosterone production can be decreased. If a man is concerned about testicular shrinkage or wants to conceive a child, there's an alternative way to replace testosterone.

Luteinizing hormone (LH), which is produced in the pituitary gland is responsible for stimulating testosterone production in the testicles. Another hormone called *human chorionic gonadotropin* (HCG) can be used as an LH mimic. When prescribed as an injection, HCG stimulates testosterone production in the testicles. There's no feedback effect to dampen the body's natural testosterone production.

HCG may be used to try to raise testosterone production in younger men whose levels are low but who want to maintain their fertility. Some doctors will give a combination of bioidentical testosterone and HCG—a weekly injection of testosterone and twice-weekly HCG, for example. Not all men's testes will respond to HCG therapy.

How to replace testosterone

Testosterone is available only by prescription. It's offered as an injection, or in a gel or patch that's applied to the skin. Testosterone pellets—which are about the size of a grain of rice—are also available. Each mode of administration has its pros and cons, but injections and pellets have seemed to work best for most men I see as patients.

Oral testosterone is almost never used in andropausal men. Although it will reliably raise testosterone levels, a very high dose of testosterone is needed to get the necessary amount through the first-pass processing by the liver. This can create byproducts that don't help and may hurt. Oral testosterone can cause "good" HDL cholesterol counts to fall and may end up causing liver damage.

Testosterone gel (Androgel) is applied daily to the shoulders or upper arms. It delivers a low, steady dose of testosterone through the skin, which is good for avoiding peaks and valleys that can create symptoms. Theoretically, the risk of transferring testosterone to one's partner is low as long as partners are careful not to make contact in the area where the gel was applied until it's completely dry. In my practice, however, this isn't the case. I've had many female patients turn up with sky-high testosterone when their partners were using Androgel. They've had symptoms like acne and growth of body hair. These were couples who told me they were being extra careful not to transfer the gel to the female partner!

The gel is much more expensive than other modes of administration—about three times the cost of injectable testosterone.

Testosterone patches (Androderm, Testoderm TTS) are applied daily. Androderm goes on the skin of the back, arm, abdomen, or upper thigh; Testoderm is applied to the scrotum. Patches can keep testosterone levels fairly even, and there's no risk of transfer to a female partner, but they can cause a rash in some users.

Testosterone injections (Andro LA 200, Delatestryl, Depandro 100, Depo-Testosterone, testosterone cypionate, testosterone enanthate) are given every one to two weeks. I teach my male patients how to inject themselves at home. With injections, there are some peaks and valleys that can cause side effects or re-emergence of andropausal symptoms, but more frequent injections of smaller amounts help keep levels constant.

Testosterone pellets (Testopel) are rice-grain-sized pellets that are inserted through a small incision. Once the man's doctor inserts it, the site takes a few days to heal. The pellet then slowly leaches testosterone into the body over a period of three to six months. When andropausal symptoms begin to return, it's time to insert another pellet.

Testosterone delivered in pellet form doesn't convert to DHT or estrogen as readily as testosterone delivered in other ways. The downside is that if testosterone goes too high with the pellet, it can't be removed; we just need to wait it out. Dose can be adjusted on the next insertion.

Side effects of too much testosterone

A skilled physician who is experienced with hormone replacement will do all he or she can to avoid giving too much—they'll start low and give more if levels don't go into the optimal range—but it's possible that a man will end up getting too much at some point. Here are a few of the symptoms or side effects men *might* experience with testosterone replacement, particularly if the dose is too high:

- Acne
- Bitter or strange taste in mouth
- Gum or mouth irritation, pain or swelling
- Extremely high sex drive or prolonged erections (priapism)
- Hair loss on head, excessive hair growth elsewhere
- Headache
- Fluid retention
- Nausea/vomiting
- Oily skin
- Rash

About 10 percent of men who replace testosterone have a rise in *hematocrit*, or blood cell count. The theoretical risk of this is a slight increase in the risk of stroke, which has not really been seen in the literature. Men who have this side effect can reduce hematocrit by giving blood once a month.

Communication and Relationship Challenges

Even when both partners achieve hormone balance, relationship issues and communication problems can get in the way of a satisfying sex life. In Chapter 12, I described a helpful form of therapy, Imago Therapy, that has helped many couples to overcome these kinds of obstacles. Here, I'd like to address another point that can help remove obstacles to intimacy: the fact that men and women tend to communicate differently and to expect different things from their partners.

This is a concept that's gotten a lot of play in pop psychology. John Gray, Ph.D.'s "Mars and Venus" books are all about how men are from Mars and women are from Venus—how their needs and expectations are different. One example Gray gives: women value daily, small expressions of love and commitment while men think they can make one big expression and have it last a while. In other words, if a man gives his partner a nice vacation, she feels loved and attended to; but he thinks that when they get home, that vacation should fulfill her need for love and attention for a while. She, on the other hand doesn't care about the size or cost of the gesture—she wants them *often*. "Instead of giving her two dozen roses," Gray advises, "give her one rose every day!"

This is only one of the many ways in which men and women differ. Deborah Tannen, Ph.D., a psychologist and communication expert, writes about the ways in which communication impacts relationships. Men and women in conversation, she writes in her book *You Just Don't Understand: Men and Women In Conversation* (William Morrow & Co., 1990), are after two different things. For men, conversation is about *doing*. It's about figuring out your own status in a group or in a pairing and about maintaining or improving that status. Men tend to take a problem-solving orientation in conversation. For women, conversation is a way to create intimacy, not to solve problems. Even if they're complaining, they feel like they're creating closeness; they aren't looking to solve anything. In conversation, men end up feeling like their partners complain or talk too much without actually wanting to fix any of their issues, and women end up feeling like they haven't been heard or heartfully communicated with.

It can truly feel, to each partner, as though they're speaking different languages—or, as John Gray suggests, like they're from different planets! That expectation of perfect, seamless, effortless relationship that many people have when they first commit to a marriage almost never seems to bear out over years and decades. And the truth is that we can use our difficulties to learn more about and become closer to our partners—as long as we're willing to seek help with our communication skills when we hit an impasse.

Help can come in many forms. Books like John Gray's or the others listed below have helped many couples to better understand and work through the relationship problems that make life less than joyous and make sexual intimacy difficult. Choose one or a few and read them together.

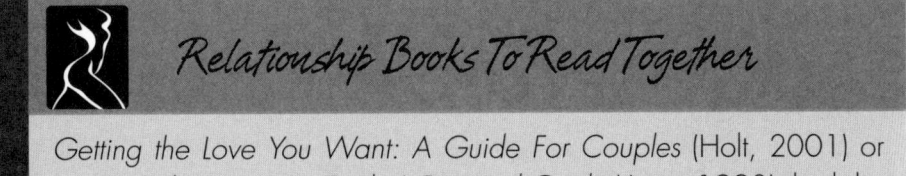

Relationship Books To Read Together

Getting the Love You Want: A Guide For Couples (Holt, 2001) or *Keeping the Love You Find: A Personal Guide* (Atria, 1993), both by Harville Hendrix, creator of Imago Therapy

I Need Your Love – Is that True? How to Stop Seeking Love, Approval, and Appreciation and Start Finding Them Instead by Byron Katie (Three Rivers Press, 2006). Katie Byron's "The Work" applied to relationships can be powerfully transformative.

Why Marriages Succeed Or Fail: and How You Can Make Yours Last (Simon & Schuster, 2001) by John Gottman, Ph.D., or *10 Lessons to Transform Your Marriage: America's Love Lab Experts Share Their Strategies For Strengthening Your Relationship* (Three Rivers Press, 2007) by John Gottman, Ph.D., Julie Schwartz Gottman and Joan Declaire. Dr. Gottman and his wife Julie run a research laboratory in Seattle called the "Love Lab," where they've been doing research on couples' communication for many years. Their books and methods are all based on this research.

Conscious Loving: The Journey to Co-Commitment (Bantam, 1992) by Gay Hendricks, Ph.D., and Kathlyn Hendricks, Ph.D. The Hendricks' methods for establishing trust and open communication are a bit more spiritually based than the methods described by Hendrix and Gottman. Their books and workshops have helped many couples create a whole new way of relating to each other.

Men Are From Mars, Women Are From Venus: the Classic Guide to Understanding the Opposite Sex (Harper, 2004) or *Mars and Venus Together Forever: Relationship Skills For Lasting Love* (Harper, 2005) by John Gray, Ph.D. These books are cute, simple and funny and have sold hundreds of thousands of copies.

How to Be an Adult in Relationships: The Five Keys to Mindful Loving by David Richo (Shambhala, 2002). This book interweaves Buddhist principles with psychology to help each partner become better at relationship.

Mating In Captivity: Unlocking Erotic Intelligence (Harper Collins, 2006) by Esther Perel, Ph.D. This book is about an interesting notion: that too much intimacy can stifle sexual desire, and that creating healthy distance between partners can actually help foster a better sexual connection.

Lots of other books and teachers are out there. Modern relationship is complicated; why not take advantage of all that expertise to learn simple ways to improve your most important relationship?

One way of approaching relationship repair might work better for you and your partner than another. Maybe each of you will find a different approach to bring to each other. The important part is that each partner wants to do whatever's necessary to make the relationship happier and healthier for both. Workshops, professional sex or relationship therapy or coaching, and spiritual practices like yoga can also help partnerships to evolve and deepen.

So: what if it *is* him and not you? It's a trick question, really. It's never just him, or just you. Adjusting hormones, healing sexual dysfunctions, eating well, being mindful and working on the relationship are almost always a team proposition in long-term partnerships. As each of you does what you can to optimize health and libido, you can bring the gifts of all of this to each other.

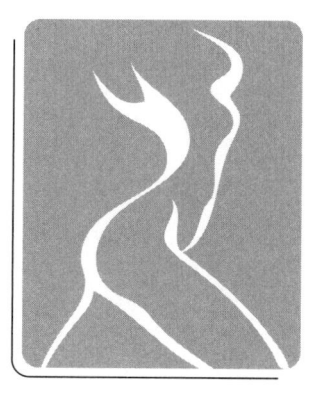

RESOURCES

Jennifer Landa M.D.
www.drjenniferlanda.com

Virginia Hopkins
www.virginiahopkinstestkits.com (test kits, books, articles)
www.virginiahopkinshealthwatch.com (blog)

BodyLogicMD
www.bodylogicmd.com

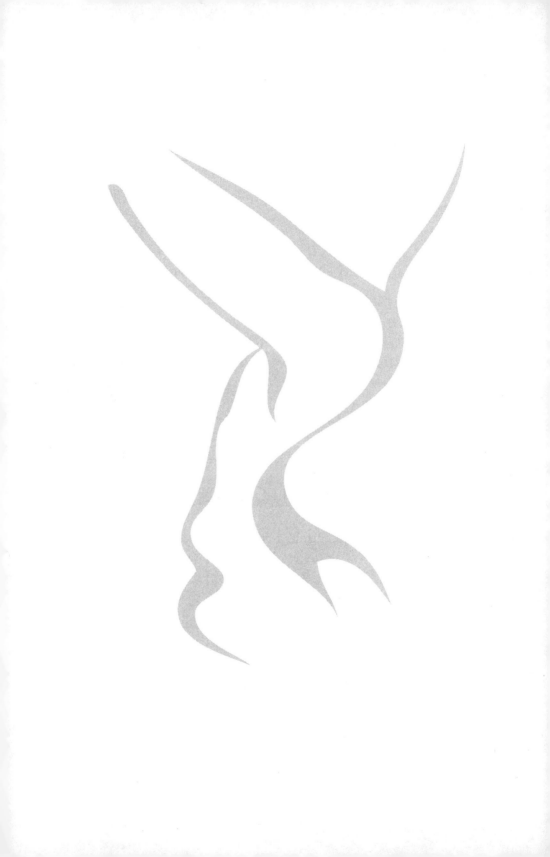

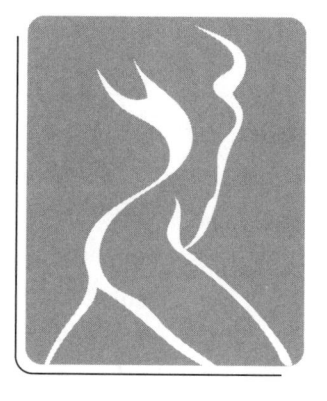

GLOSSARY

Adrenal glands: Two walnut-sized and shaped glands that sit just above the kidneys, behind the lower back ribs. They produce dozens of hormones and other substances, the most familiar of which are the cortisols and the adrenalines.

Amenorrhoea: The absence of a menstrual period in a premenopausal woman

Androgenic: Producing masculine characteristics

Androstenedione: An androgenic (masculinizing) hormone

Anovulatory: Suspension or cessation of ovulation

Aromatization: Conversion of a cyclic organic compound to phenol-like form, such as the conversion of testosterone to estrogen in body fat

BHRT: Stands for "bioidentical hormone replacement therapy"

Bioidentical: Identical to what is made by the human body

Blastoderm: The early mass of cells produced by cleavage of a fertilized ovum

Carcinogen: Any cancer-producing substance

Conjugated: In biochemistry, one compound combined with another, such as combining estrogen in chemical contraceptives and HRT with another molecule(s) to create a hormone not found in nature so that it can be patented

Corpus luteum: Small yellow glandular mass in the ovary formed by an ovarian follicle after ovulation (release of its egg [ovum])

Corticosteroids: Hormones produced by the adrenal cortex

Dysmenorrhoea: Painful menstruation

Endocrine: Refers to organs (glands) that secrete substances such as hormones such as the ovaries, testes and thyroid gland

Endogenous: Developing or originating within the body

Endometriosis: The abnormal growth of endometrial cells that normally line the uterus, outside of the uterus, usually in the abdominal cavity

Endometrium: The inner lining of the uterus

Enzyme: An organic compound, usually a protein, capable of producing a change in some substrate for which it is often specific

Episiotomy: A cut made in the perineum during childbirth to widen the opening of the vagina to avoid tearing during delivery

Estrone, estradiol and estriol: Female sex hormones known collectively as estrogens, they are primarily responsible for the growth of female characteristics in puberty and regulating the menstrual cycle. They are made primarily in the ovaries but also from androstenedione in fat cells, muscle cells, and skin even after menopause.

Exogenous: Originating outside of the body

Fibroid (uterine): A benign (non-cancerous) fibrous tumor in the uterus, very common in premenopausal women and can cause heavy bleeding, the leading cause of hysterectomy

Follicle: A very small excretory or secretory sac or gland, e.g., the ovarian follicle that produces the ovum

Genital: Having to do with the external and internal organs of reproduction, such as the uterus, vagina, vulva, labia, cervix and clitoris

HRT: Stands for "hormone replacement therapy" and is usually used to refer to conventional medicine's synthetic combination of Premarin and Provera (PremPro), but can really refer to any type of supplemental hormone use

Hysterectomy: Surgical removal of the uterus

Laparoscopy: A minimally invasive surgery often used to remove fibroids or ovaries, involving a small incision in the abdomen

through which an instrument called a laparoscope is inserted

Libido: The sex drive

Luteinizing: Refers to maturation of ovarian follicles for ovulation after which the follicle become the corpus luteum producing progesterone

Menopause: Officially begins one year after a woman's last menstrual period

Metabolism: The biochemical process of living organisms by which substances are produced and energy is made available to the organism

Microgram (mcg): One-millionth $(10\text{-}6)$ of a gram

Milligram (mg): One-thousandth $(10\text{-}3)$ of a gram

Nanogram (ng): One-billionth $(10\text{-}9)$ of a gram

Oocytes: The cell that produces the ovum

Oophorectomy: Surgical removal of an ovary or ovaries

Oral: By mouth, such as a pill taken by mouth

Ovary: One of two glands located above the uterus in females responsible for releasing estrogen, progesterone and testosterone, as well as an egg each month in menstruating women

Perimenopausal: Refers to the time preceding menopause when hormone changes and fluctuations are occurring and overall hormone levels are falling

Perineum: The skin between the vaginal opening and the anus

Pregnenolone: A hormone synthesized from cholesterol by mitochondria of all the cells of the body (except red blood cells), this molecule is the precursor to all steroid hormones.

Premenopausal: The twenty years or so prior to menopause

Steroid: Group name for compounds based on cholesterol molecule, e.g., sex hormones and corticosteroids

Suppository: Medication in soft, solid form designed for insertion into the rectum or vagina, where it dissolves

Transdermal: Through the skin, such as a progesterone or estrogen cream applied to the skin in a cream, gel or patch

Troche: A lozenge or candy containing medication that is held in the mouth to dissolve

Xeno-: Combining form, meaning strange, or denoting relationship to foreign material such as xenoestrogens, which are pollutants and toxins with estrogen-like effects in the body

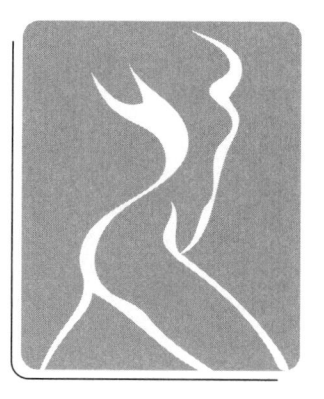

REFERENCES

Chapter 2 References

American Economic Journal: Economic Policy 2009, 1:2, 190-225.

Barkow, Jerome H, Cosmides, Leda, and Tooby, John (editors). *The Adapted Mind: Evolutionary Psychology and the Generation of Culture* (Oxford University Press, USA 1995).

Taylor, Timothy. *The Prehistory of Sex: Four Million Years of Sexual Culture* (Bantam Books, 1997).

Whipps, Heather, "A Brief History of Human Sex," **www.livescience.com/health/060627_sex_history.html**.

Chapter 3 References

"What are the key statistics about cervical cancer?" American Cancer Society website, **www.cancer.org/docroot/CRI/content/CRI_2_4_1X_ What_are_the_key_statistics_for_cervical_cancer_8.asp;** accessed 2/3/10.

Ackerman, Diane. *A Natural History of the Senses.* (Vintage Books, New York, NY: 1990)

Deane Juhan, *Job's Body: A Handbook for Bodywork*. Station Hill Press, Barrytown NY:1987.

Grafenberg, Ernst, "The Role of Urethra in Female Orgasm," Journal of Sexology, 1950.

Gravina GL, Brandetti F, Martini P et al, "Measurement of the thickness of the urethrovaginal space in women with or without vaginal orgasms." *J Sex Med* 5:610.

Jain S, Mills PJ, "Biofield therapies: helpful or full of hype? A best-evidence synthesis," *Int J Behav Med* 2009 Oct 24.

McClintock MK, "On the nature of mammalian and human pheromones." *Ann N Y Acad Sci*, Nov. 1998 30; 855: 390-2.

Sprinkle, Annie. "Seven Types of Female Orgasm," **www.anniesprinkle. org/html/writings/7_types_org.html**.

Wedekind C, Furi S. "Body odor preferences in men and women: Do they aim for specific MHC combinations or simply heterozygoity?" *Proc R Soc Lond B Biol Sci*. Oct. 1997: 264 (137); 1471-9.

Chapter 4 References

Apter D, "Serum steroids and pituitary hormones in female puberty: a partly longitudinal study," *Clinical Endocrinology* 1980 Feb; 12 (2): 107–20.

Arem, Ridha MD, *The Thyroid Solution*, Ballantine Books, New York, NY:1999.

Bolaji II, et al, "Assessment of bioavailability of oral micronized progesterone using a salivary progesterone enzymeimmunoassay," *Gynecol Endocrinol* 1993;7:101-10.

Bolton JL, et al, "Role of quinoids in estrogen carcinogenesis," *Chem Res Toxicol* 1998;11(10):1113-27.

Bradlow HL, et al, "2-hydroxyestrone: the 'good' estrogen," *J Endocrinol* 1996;150 Suppl:S259-65.

Chatterton et al, "Characteristics of salivary profiles of oestradiol and progesterone in premenopausal women," J Endocrinol 2005;186:77-84.

Fowke JH, et al, "Brassica vegetable consumption shifts estrogen metabolism in healthy postmenopausal women," *Cancer Epidemiol Biomarkers Prev* 2000;9(8):773-9.

Gann et al, "Saliva as a medium for investigating intra- and interindividual differences in sex hormone levels in premenopausal women," *Cancer Epidemiol Biomarkers Prev* 2001;10:59-64.

Gozansky WS, Lynn JS, Laudenslager ML, et al, "Salivary cortisol determined by enzyme immunoassay is preferable to serum total cortisol for assessment of dynamic hypothalamic-pituitary-adrenal axis activity," *Clin Endocrinol* 2005;63:336-41.

Haggans CJ, et al. "Effect of flaxseed consumption on urinary estrogen metabolites in postmenopausal women," *Nutr Cancer* 1999;33(2):188-95.

Huang Z, et al, "16-alpha-hydroxylation of estrone by human cytochrome P4503A4/5," *Carcinogenesis* 1998;19(5):867-72.

Lee, John R. MD, and Virginia Hopkins, *Dr. John Lee's Hormone Balance Made Simple: The Essential How-To Guide to Symptoms, Dosage, Timing and More*, Warner Wellness, New York, NY:2006.

Lee, John R., MD, and Virginia Hopkins, *What Your Doctor May Not Tell You About Menopause: The Breakthrough Book on Natural Hormone Balance*, Grand Central Publishing, New York, NY: 2004.

Lee, John R., MD, Virginia Hopkins and Jesse Hanley, MD, *What Your Doctor May Not Tell You About PREmenopause: Balance Your Hormones and Your Life From Thirty to Fifty*, Grand Central Publishing, New York, NY: 2005.

Leonetti et al, "Transdermal progesterone cream as an alternative progestin in hormone therapy," *Altern Ther Health Med* 2005;11:36-8.

Muti P, et al, "Estrogen metabolism and risk of breast cancer: a prospective study of the 2:16 alpha-hydroxyestrone ratio in premenopausal and postmenopausal women," *Epidemiology* 2000;11(6):635-40.

Chapter 5 References

Abraham GE, "Ovarian and adrenal contribution to peripheral androgens during the menstrual cycle," 1974 *J Clin Endocrinol Metab* 39:340–346.

Adashi EY, "The climacteric ovary as a functional gonadotropin-driven androgen-producing gland" *Fertil Steril* 1994;62:20-27.

Al-Azzawi F, Bitzer J, Brandenburg U et al, "Therapeutic options for postmenopausal female sexual dysfunction," *Climacteric* Apr 2010, Vol. 13, No. 2, Pages 103-120.

Davis SR, Moreau M, Kroll R et al, "Testosterone for low libido in postmenopausal women not taking estrogen," *N Eng J Med* 2008 Nov 6;359(19):2005-17.

Davis SR, Humberstone A, Milne RW, Evans AM, "Measurement of serum total testosterone levels after administration of testosterone can underestimate the amount of testosterone that has been absorbed," 2003 Proceedings of The Endocrine Society's 85th Annual Meeting, Philadelphia.

Eckardstein A, Wu FC, "Testosterone and atherosclerosis," *Growth Horm IGF Res* 2003 Aug;13 Suppl A:S72-84.

Judd HL, Judd GE, Lucas WE, Yen SS, "Endocrine function of the postmenopausal ovary: concentration of androgens and estrogens in ovarian and peripheral vein blood," *J Clin Endocrinol Meta* 1974;39:1020-1024.

Khatibi A, Agardh CD, Shakir YA, "Could androgens protect middle-aged women from cardiovascular events? A population-based study of Swedish women: The Women's Health in the Lund Area (WHILA) Study," *Climacteric* 2007 Oct;10(5):386-92.

Kingsberg SA, Simon JA, Goldstein I, "The current outlook for testosterone in the management of hypoactive sexual desire disorder in postmenopausal women," *J Sex Med* 2008 Sep 2;5 Suppl 4:182-93; quiz 193.

Klee GG, Heser DW, "Techniques to measure testosterone in the elderly," *Mayo Clinic Proceedings* 75:S19-S25, 2000.

Laughlin G, Barrett-Connor E, Kritz-Silverstein D, Von Muhlen D, "Hysterectomy, oophorectomy, and endogenous sex hormone levels in older women: the Rancho Bernardo Study," 2000 *J Clin Endocrinol Metab.* 85:645–651.

Ness RB, Albano JD, McTiernan A, Cauley JA, "Influence of estrogen plus testosterone supplementation on breast cancer," *Arch Intern Med* 2009 Jan 12;169(1):41-6.

Panay N, Al-Azzawi F, Bouchard C et al, "Testosterone treatment of HSDD in naturally menopausal women: the ADORE study," *Climacteric* 2010 Apr;13(2):121-31.

Shufelt CL, Braunstein GD, "Safety of testosterone use in women," *Maturitas* 2009 May 20;63(1):63-6.

Vermeulen A, Verdonck L, Kaufman M, "A critical evaluation of simple methods for the estimation of free testosterone in serum," *J Clin Endocrinol Metab* 84:3666-3672, 1999.

Chapter 6 References

Chen KK and Chiu JH. Effect of Epimedium brevicornum Maxim extract on elicitation of penile erection in the rat. *Urology.* 67.3 (2006):631-5.

Cohen AJ, Bartlik B, "Ginkgo biloba for antidepressant-induced sexual dysfunction," *J Sex Marital Ther* 1998 Apr-Jun;24(2):139-43.

Ito TY, Polan ML, Whipple B, Trant AS. "The enhancement of female sexual function with ArginMax, a nutritional supplement, among women differing in sexual status." *J Sex Marital Ther* 2006 Oct-Dec;32(5):369-78.

Ito TY, Trant AS, Polan ML. "A double-blind placebo-controlled study of ArginMax, a nutritional supplement for enhancement of female sexual function." *J Sex Marital Ther* 2001 Oct-Dec;27(5):541-9.

Oh MH et al. Screening of Korean herbal medicines used to improve cognitive function for anti-cholinesterase activity. *Phytomedicine.* 11.6 (2004):544-8.

Murphy LL, Lee TJ, "Ginseng, sex behavior, and nitric oxide," *Ann NY Acad Sci* 2002 May;962:372-7.

Schulman SP, Becker LC, Kass DA et al, "L-arginine therapy in acute myocardial infarction: the Vascular Interaction With Age in Myocardial Infarction (VINTAGE MI) randomized clinical trial," *JAMA.* 2006 Jan 4.

Shamloul Rany MD, Natural Aphrodisiacs (Review), *J Sex Med* 2010;7:39-49.

Wheatley D, "Triple-blind, placebo-controlled trial of Ginkgo biloba in sexual dysfunction due to antidepressant drugs," *Hum Psychopharmacol* 2004 Dec;19(8):545-8.

Zhang CZ et al. In vitro estrogenic activities of Chinese medicinal plants traditionally used for the management of menopausal symptoms. *Journal of Ethnopharmacology.* 98.3 (2005):295-300.

Chapter 7 References

Adverse Drug Reactions Advisory Committee, "Simvastatin and adverse endocrine effects in men," *Aust Adverse Drug Reactions Bull* 1995;14:10.

Baton R, "SSRI-associated sexual dysfunction," *Am J Psychiatr* 2006;163: 1504-1509.

Bonakdar RA, Guarneri E, "Coenzyme Q10," *Am Fam Physician* 2005 Sep 15;72(6):1065-70.

Boyles, Salynn, "Birth control, HRT and sex drive: monkey study may help explain why synthetic hormones affect libido," *WebMD Health News*, **www.webmd.com/sex/birth-control/features/no-more-periods?page=4.** Accessed 5/8/10.

Breggin, Peter R., *Brain-Disabling Treatments In Psychiatry: Drugs, Electroshock, and the Psychopharmaceutical Complex*, 2nd Ed. Springer Publishing Company, New York, NY:2008.

Bruckert E, et al, "Men treated with hypolipidaemic drugs complain more frequently of erectile dysfunction," *J Clin Pharm Ther* 1996; 21(2):89-94.

Elias PK, et al, "Serum cholesterol and cognitive performance in the Framingham Heart Study," *Psychosom Med.* 2005 Jan-Feb;67(1):24–30.

Golomb BA, "Impact of statin adverse events in the elderly," *Expert Opin Drug Saf* 2005;4(3):389–397.

Jackson G, "Simvastatin and impotence," *BMJ* 1997;315:31.

Koo SI, Noh SK, "Green tea as inhibitor of the intestinal absorption of lipids: potential mechanism for its lipid-lowering effect," *J Nutr Biochem* 2007;18(3):179-83.

L de Graff, et al, "Is decreased libido associated with the use of HMG-CoA-reductase-inhibitors?" *B J Clin Pharmacol* 2004;58(3):326-8.

Lee W, Min WK, Chun S, et al, "Long-term effects of green tea ingestion on atherosclerotic biological markers in smokers," *Clin Biochem* 2005 Jan 1;38(1):84-87.

Malatesta, V.J., Pollack, R.H., Crotty, T.D., et al. "Acute Alcohol Intoxication and the Female Orgasmic Response." *Journal of Sex Research* 1982;
Volume 18:1-17.

Miller NS, Gold MS, "The human sexual response and alcohol and drugs," *J Subst Abuse Treat* 1988; 5:171-7.

Mindell, Earl L., R.Ph., Ph.D. and Virginia Hopkins, MA. *Prescription Alternatives: Hundreds of Safe, Natural, Prescription-Free Remedies to Restore and Maintain Your Health.* 4th ed. McGraw-Hill, New York, NY: 2009.

Muldoon MF, et al, "Randomized trial of the effects of simvastatin on cognitive functioning in hypercholesterolemic adults," *Am J Med* 2004;117(11):823–829.

Onland-Moren NC, Peeters PH, Van der Schouw YT, et al, "Alcohol and endogenous sex steroid levels in postmenopausal women: a cross-sectional study," *J Clin Endocrinol Metab* 2004;90(3):1414-1419.

Panzer C, Wise S, Fantini G, et al, "Impact of oral contraceptives on sex hormone-binding globulin and androgen levels: a retrospective study in women with sexual dysfunction," *J Sex Med* 2006 Jan;3(1):104-13.

Pfrieger FW, "Role of cholesterol in synapse formation and function," *Biochim Biophys Acta* 2003 Mar 10;1610(2):271–280.

Physicians' Desk Reference, 61st Edition. Montvale, NJ: Thompson PDR; 2007.

Rizvi K, et al, "Do lipid lowering drugs cause erectile dysfunction? A systematic review," *Family Practice* 2002;19 (1):95-8.

Sarkola T, Fukunaga T, Makisalo H, et al, "Acute effect of alcohol on androgens in premenopausal women," *Alcohol and Alcoholism* 2000;35(1):84-90.

Saul, Stephanie, "Sleep Drugs Found Only Mildly Effective, But Wildly Popular," *New York Times*, October 23, 2007.

Stomati M, Hartmann B, Spinetti A, et al, "Effects of hormonal replacement therapy on plasma sex hormone-binding globulin, androgen and insulin-like growth factor-1 levels in postmenopausal women," *J Endocrinol Invest* 1996 Sep;19(8):535-41.

Tattelman E, "Health effects of garlic," *Am Fam Physician* 2005 Jul 1;72(01):103-6.

Thavendiranathan P, Bagai A, Brookhart MI, et al, "Primary prevention of cardiovascular disease with statin therapy: a meta-analysis of randomized controlled trials," *Arch Intern Med* 2006 Nov 27;166(21):2307-13.

Wider B, Pittler MH, Thompson-Coon J et al, "Artichoke leaf for treating hypercholesterolemia," *Cochrane Databases Syst Rev* 2009 Oct 7;4:CD003335.

Chapter 11 References

Bloch M, Daly RC, Rubinow DR, "Endocrine factors in the etiology of postpartum depression," *Compr Psychiatry* 2003 May-Jun;44(3):234-46.

Bloch M, et al, "Effects of gonadal steroids in women with a history of postpartum depression," *Am J Psychiatry* 2000 Jun;157(6):924-30.

Chrousos GP, Torpy DJ, Gold PW, "Interactions between the hypothalamic-pituitary-adrenal axis and the female reproductive system: clinical implications," *Ann Intern Med* 1998 Aug 1;129(3):229-40;

LaMarre AK, Paterson LQ, Gorzalka BB, "Maternal sexual functioning: a review," *The Canadian Journal of Human Sexuality*, 2003 Sep 22.

Interview with Bob Gottesman, **www.virginiahopkinstestkits.com/ depresshor.html**, accessed 4/14/10.

Chapter 12 References

Blumenthal M, Goldberg A, Brinckman J, eds. *Herbal Medicine: Expanded Commission E Monographs.* Newton, MA: Lippincott Williams & Wilkins; 2000:62–64.

Brooks JD, Ward WE, Lewis JE, et al, "Supplementation with flax seed alters estrogen metabolism in postmenopausal women to a greater extent than does supplementation with an equal amount of soy," *Am J Clin Nutr* 2004 Feb;79(2):318-25.

Coates P, Blackman M, Cragg G, et al., eds. *Encyclopedia of Dietary Supplements.* New York, NY: Marcel Dekker; 2005:95–103.

Gentile GP, Kaufman SC, Helbig DW, "Is there any evidence for a post-tubal sterilization syndrome?" *Fertil Steril* 1998 Feb;69(2):179-86.

Kohler TS, Fazili AA, Brannigan RE, "Putative health risks associated with vasectomy," *Urol Clin North Am* 2009 Aug;36(3):337-45.

Peterson HB, Jeng G, Folger SG, et al, "The risk of menstrual abnormalities after tubal sterilization. U.S. Collaborative Review of Sterilization Working Group," *N Engl J Med* 2000 Dec 7;343(23):1681-7.

Peterson HB, "Sterilization," *Obstet Gynecol* 2008 Jan;111(1):189-203.

Higdon JV, Delage B, Williams DE, et al, "Cruciferous vegetables and human cancer risk: epidemiologic evidence and mechanistic basis," *Pharmacol Res* 2007 March;55(3):224-236.

Herr I, Büchler MW, "Dietary constituents of broccoli and other cruciferous vegetables: implications for prevention and therapy of cancer," *Cancer Treat Rev* 2010 Feb 19. Epub ahead of print.

Sturgeon SR, Heersink JL, Volpe SL, et al, "Effect of dietary flaxseed on serum levels of estrogens and androgens in postmenopausal women," *Nutr Cancer* 2008;60(5):612-8.

Chapter 13 References
Weiderpass E, Adami HO, Baron JA et al, "Risk of Endometrial Cancer Following Estrogen Replacement With and Without Progestins," *JNCI* Vol. 91, No. 13, July 7, 1999.

Jick H, Walker AM, Rothman KJ, "The Epidemic of Endometrial Cancer: A Commentary," *AJPH* March 1980, Vol. 70, No. 3.

Chapter 15 References
Amore M, Scarlatti F, Quarta AL, et al, "Partial androgen deficiency, depression and testosterone treatment in aging men," *Aging Clin Exp Res* 2009 Feb;
21(1):1-8.

Anawalt BD, Merriam GR, "Neuroendocrine aging in men: andropause and somatopause," *Endocrinol Metab Clin* North Am 2001 Sep;30(3):647-69.

Eckardstein A, Wu FC, "Testosterone and atherosclerosis," *Growth Horm IGF Res* 2003 Aug;13 Suppl A:S72-84.

Eskelinen SI, Vahlberg TJ, Isoaho RE, et al, "Associations of sex hormone concentrations with health and life satisfaction in elderly men," *Endocr Pract* 2007 Nov-Dec;13(7):743-9.

McCarthy, Barry, and Emily McCarthy. *Rekindling Desire: A Step-By-Step Program to Help Low-Sex and No-Sex Marriages.* Taylor & Francis Books, New York, NY: 2003.

Nettleship JE, Jones RD, Channer KS, et al, "Testosterone and coronary artery disease," *Front Horm Res* 2009;37:91-107.

Nicolosi A, Laumann EO, Glasser DB, et al, "Sexual behavior and sexual dysfunctions after age 40: the global study of sexual attitudes and behaviors," *Urology* 2004 Nov;64(5):991-7.

Ohl DA, Quallich SA, "Clinical hypogonadism and androgen replacement therapy: an overview," **www.medscape.com/ viewarticle/543997_7.** Accessed 5/24/10.

Rosano GM, Sheiban I, Massaro R, et al, "Low testosterone levels are associated with coronary artery disease in male patients with angina," *Int J Impot Res* 2007 Mar-Apr;19(2):176-82. Epub 2006 Aug 31.

Seliger, Susan, "Loss of libido in men: why men lose interest in sex – and 8 tips to rekindle desire." **www.webmd.com/sex-relationships/features/ loss-of-libido-in-men.** Accessed 5/25/10.

Tostain JL, Blanc F, "Testosterone deficiency: a common, unrecognized syndrome," *Nat Clin Pract Urol* 2008 Jul;5(7):388-96.

Vandenput L, Ohlsson C, "Sex steroid metabolism in the regulation of bone health in men," *J Steroid Biochem Mol Biol* 2010 Mar 31.

Webb CM, Collins P, "Testosterone and coronary artery disease in men," *Maturitas* 2010 May 4.

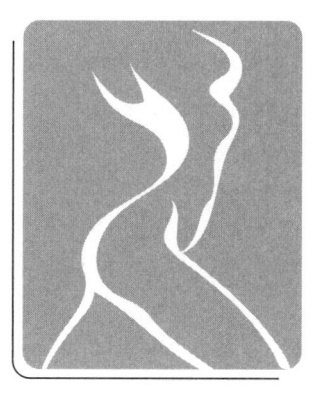

AUTHOR BIOGRAPHIES

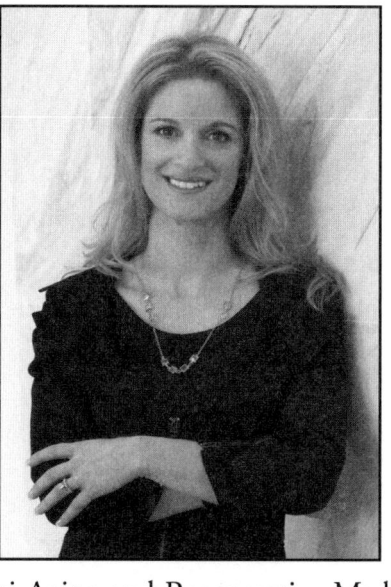

Dr. Jennifer Landa is a fortysomething wife, mother, physician and speaker whose energetic, upbeat and straight-forward style has made her a favorite of women seeking health solutions, from fatigue, PMS, and low sex drive, to baby blues, hot flashes and menopausal mood swings.

After a decade working as a traditional OB/GYN, Dr. Landa realized she wanted more—for her patients and herself. She spent two years becoming certified in Anti-Aging and Regenerative Medicine, with an emphasis on hormones and nutrition. She specializes in helping women restore their energy and their sex lives, and is the Chief Medical Officer of BodyLogicMD. Dr. Landa regularly speaks to physician and lay audiences on the subject of female sexuality and hormone balance.

Practicing MD, author, blogger and triathelete, Dr. Landa also serves as volunteer faculty at UCF Medical College and performs volunteer gynecologic care at a local women's clinic. She earned her medical degree from Albany Medical College of Union University in Albany, NY in 1996, and completed her internship and residency at Beth Israel Medical Center in NYC, where she was distinguished as the Administrative Chief Resident in OB/GYN.

Dr. Landa lives in Orlando, FL with her husband and two children.

For more information about Dr. Landa, visit her website at **www.drjenniferlanda.com**.

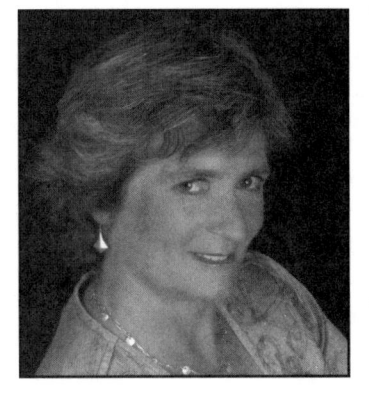

Virginia Hopkins has been a writer and editor since she graduated from Yale University in 1976. She is co-author of the highly successful "*What Your Doctor May Not Tell You...*" books with Dr. John Lee. She is also co-author of the best-selling book *Prescription Alternatives*. Hopkins is currently the author/editor of a popular newsletter and website, the Virginia Hopkins Health Watch.

For more information about Virginia Hopkins, visit her website at **www.virginiahopkinshealthwatch.com**.

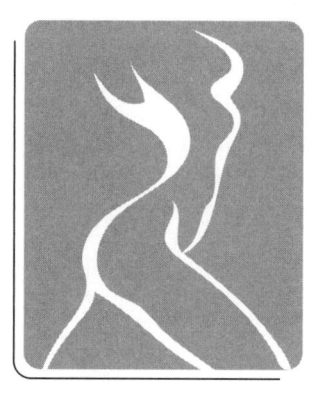

INDEX

E

Erectile dysfunction, 277, 278, 25, 95, 100, 104, 118, 153, 181, 192, 229, 242-244, 12

Erotica, 41, 178, 179, 190, 193, 194, 210, 11

Estradiol, 53, 65, 81, 85, 100, 110, 113, 114, 127, 232, 268

Estriol, 53, 65, 81, 114, 268, 14

Estrogen, 272-275, 279, 280, 42, 45, 47, 50, 53, 58, 62-73, 75-82, 84, 85, 88-91, 100, 108, 111-114, 120, 132, 135, 163, 177, 198, 201, 204, 205, 212-220, 226, 227, 231-234, 240, 243, 244, 251, 256, 259, 267, 268, 270, 8, 11

Estrogen dominance, 67-71, 73, 76, 77, 81, 82, 85, 88, 91, 163, 205, 212-219, 227, 240, 8, 11

F

Fitness, 32, 148, 209, 232, 2

G

G-spot, 49, 53, 54, 58, 192, 233, 15, 8

H

Heart disease, 24, 86, 87, 91, 95, 119, 133, 137, 153, 169, 170, 228, 252, 9

Hendrix, 220-223, 262

Herbs, 93-96, 99, 105, 106, 117, 125, 134, 137, 151, 245, 9

High blood pressure, 22, 96, 102, 104, 116, 120, 132, 245, 246, 250

History, 271, 279, 26, 30-35, 193, 217, 222, 245, 254, 7

Hormone replacement therapy, 24, 45, 79, 113, 146, 185, 267, 269

Hot flashes, 51, 57, 78, 79, 225, 228, 232, 238, 240, 12

HRT, 277, 24, 79, 80, 111, 114, 226, 228, 253, 268, 269

Hypertension, 114-117, 245, 9

Hysterectomy, 275, 40, 52, 55-58, 62, 84, 216, 225, 226, 269, 8

I

Incontinence, 52, 53, 79, 86, 187

Intercourse, painful, 64, 201

IUD, 109, 112, 113, 204, 217

K

Kegels, 187

L

Labia majora, 39, 47

Labia minora, 39, 40, 47, 48

Lubricants, 231, 248, 16

Lubricate, 47, 55

Lubrication, 26, 51, 97, 114, 127